Accidental Kindness

ALSO BY MICHAEL STEIN

FICTION

Probabilities

The White Life

The Lynching Tree

In the Age of Love

This Room Is Yours

The Rape of the Muse

NONFICTION

The Lonely Patient: How We Experience Illness

The Addict: One Patient, One Doctor, One Year

Pained: Uncomfortable Conversations about the Public's Health

Broke: Patients Talk about Money with Their Doctor

Me vs. Us: A Health Divided

Accidental Kindness

A Doctor's Notes on Empathy

MICHAEL STEIN, M.D.

THE UNIVERSITY OF NORTH CAROLINA PRESS

Chapel Hill

*This book was published with the assistance of the
Anniversary Fund of the University of North Carolina Press.*

Designed by Jamison Cockerham
Set in Scala, Professor, and American Typewriter
by codeMantra

Manufactured in the United States of America

Cover illustration: © iStock/Normform

LIBRARY OF CONGRESS CATALOGING-IN-PUBLICATION DATA
Names: Stein, Michael, 1960– author.
Title: Accidental kindness : a doctor's notes
on empathy / Michael Stein, M.D.
Description: Chapel Hill : The University
of North Carolina Press, 2022.
Identifiers: LCCN 2022017106 | ISBN 9781469671802
(cloth ; alk. paper) | ISBN 9781469671819 (pbk. ;
alk. paper) | ISBN 9781469671826 (ebook)
Subjects: LCSH: Stein, Michael, 1960– | Physician
and patient—United States. | Physicians—United
States—Conduct of life. | Kindness. | Empathy.
Classification: LCC R727.3 .S755 2022 | DDC
610.69/6—dc23/eng/20220613
LC record available at https://lccn.loc.gov/2022017106

FOR MY FATHER,

still chasing me,

AND FOR MY SONS,

kind always

It is a little facile, maybe, and certainly hard
to implement, but I'd say, as a goal in life,
you could do worse than "Try to be kinder."

George Saunders

CONTENTS

A NOTE TO THE READER

This book contains the stories of real people. They share their stories in confidence and I must honor that trust. I have changed names and genders and places, as well as physical descriptions of the speakers. In some cases, I have created composites to protect anonymity. I hope to disguise; anyone recognizable is coincidental.

Accidental Kindness

Introduction

Soon after I turned fifty, I made a mistake in my medical office and deeply hurt a patient. I said something I shouldn't have, and I knew it immediately. Beatriz had been my patient for many years, and what I said was unkind and probably unforgiveable; I certainly couldn't forgive myself. Not long after, and perhaps as a result of this first mistake, I uncharacteristically made two other small but notable errors in judgment with patients, and then another with a hospitalized patient, Mr. Kadden, whom I'd known for years. In the aftermath, I decided to take a month off from my primary care medicine practice.

I was already the author of six novels, so I began to write as a means of discovery and recovery, and as an attempt to make sense of what I had done. When I returned to doctoring, I started the long process of remorse, and over the next years I took notes on moments and experiences of kindness and unkindness, of forgiveness and unforgiveness, that occurred during my clinical hours. I thought about how my patients viewed me, which ones gave me the benefit of the doubt, which ones I had to convince about the rightness of my ideas, which ones I softened or grew tougher around. I sought medical and psychological research that might explain my feelings and behavior. I thought about my medical training. I thought about my father, who had died one night in an emergency room when I was thirteen years old—the event that drove me toward medicine but that also was at the root of my impossible need to be flawless in my medical activities and my difficulty with self-forgiveness. I wrote in search of coherence. Writing is remembering.

We will all be patients sooner or later. In an emergency, we want our doctors to be decisive, efficient, and competent, and to take on the weightiest of decisions with us and on our behalf. Most doctor visits are not emergencies, though—they are literally "primary" care; and for these routine interactions, while we still want a doctor's time, attention, and presence, we are also looking for advice and relief, safety and approval. Hurting, betrayed by our bodies, we think of chronic illness in terms of cause and condemnation, and we believe a doctor can at least partly relieve our self-blame, shame, and sense of inadequacy. We want our doctors to offer kindness under any of its many names—generosity, empathy, caring, compassion, benevolence, humanity.

Early during my first year of medical school, I completed a questionnaire that a graduate student was circulating for her thesis. Her survey included the question "Would you rather be intelligent or kind?" The answer was obvious to me and took not a second's thought: I checked "intelligent." I was, after all, beginning medical school, and intelligence was what I needed, what mattered. Looking back, the entirety of my career has been a slow understanding that I checked the wrong box.

The stories in *Accidental Kindness* confirm for patients that their doctors often do not give enough—enough touch or care or reassurance or time—and that they are right to ask for more, but also that sometimes the truth hurts patients, even if it's kindly meant. I have come to believe that kindness results from an intuition of how much truth to give at any moment, how best to share it, something I never would have guessed when I started medical school.

When I reconsider how doctors are trained and what would lead us to be kind or unkind, I wonder whether unkindness—which can be as damaging as other medical errors—is a natural outgrowth of doctors' education. Maybe some people are born kind and forgiving; certainly others have to be taught and to try harder. If kindness is the ability to bear the vulnerability of others and oneself, was I ever taught this in my years of schooling? What I learned after leaving school was that kindness, unlike the rest of medicine, must be more than received ideas and information presented in the form of approved emotions. Kindness requires a fresh response and an effort to see clearly and feel directly, even when it is impossible to predict whether and how it will be received at all.

That doctors are accused of unkindness during careers where so many situations are emotionally fraught, when they deal with so many people who are unhappy and in pain and scared, might be expected. Can doctors ever be *too* kind? Counterintuitively, empathy, the very source of kindness, may also be the source of compassion fatigue. I believe compassion can be pathological. Doctors can reach a state of reduced capacity for kindness as a result of exhaustion from absorbing the suffering of others. Preceding my rupturing visit with Beatriz, might I have anticipated my unacceptable behavior if I'd been more alert to my feelings?

Doctors are good at figuring things out, but even better at assigning blame. Patients make big messes of themselves, often caused by the conditions of their lives—the violence at home, the damaged stairs that make them fall, the cigarettes that lessen their anxiety but leave them short of breath—giving doctors plenty of opportunities to reproach, question, reprimand, castigate. Patients, ill, broken, sometimes think badly of themselves. And each day doctors must decide to blame or to be merciful. It shouldn't be a difficult choice—doctors are asked (and paid) to accept life as it presents itself and practice kindness anyway—but it is. Perhaps it is because doctors, as I've learned, carry their own forms of self-blame. Or perhaps because doctors remain unconvinced that kindness really matters. Does kindness save lives? When the skeptic demands proof, persuasive evidence is indeed hard to find.

"Kindness" is not a term used in the medical literature; it is not included in the mission statement of health care organizations. I've never heard "forgiveness" whispered in the halls of clinics or hospitals where I've worked. Yet it seems that patients know exactly what kindness feels like. At times kindness, in the form of forgiveness, seems hard for medical providers to access. Doctors live in a world of slow-motion crises, self-centered fear, and saving people. Doctors deal each day with tales of the worried, sullen, skeptical, dissipated, desperate. Sometimes we get weakened by others' troubles. Sometimes we simply stop paying attention. Sometimes we misunderstand a need. Doctors hurt patients not only with needles and catheters but also with words and terseness and errors in judgment, and patients have the right to understand why.

In *Accidental Kindness* I offer the experiences of one writer who has been a patient, and the son of patients, and also a doctor whose greatest unrecognized pleasure *is* kindness. I hope to show readers what they might expect and what might go wrong in the intimate patient-doctor interaction. I reexamine the often conflicting goals of patients and medicine. I believe kindness should not become the patient's forbidden or unrealistic expectation. Kindness and the largeness of spirit that goes with it must not be lost to doctors in the medical setting.

Five years after Beatriz, I met a doctor who'd made a different kind of mistake; I also met his injured patient, who taught me about forgiveness and the miracle of apology, given and accepted; sometimes a patient can relieve their doctor's guilt. After hearing their story, I began to awaken to the many forms kindness can take. This patient, by sharing her story, allowed me to start to forgive myself for my errors with Beatriz and Mr. Kadden. It was among the hardest things I've ever done.

Mistakes happen. For most of my life I'd harbored the belief that my father died as a result of a medical mistake. But this injured patient taught me that you can change your past—not what happened, but your emotional relationship to what happened. That is the premise of forgiveness. Forgiveness is the radical form of kindness that incorporates the past. Forgiveness is messy, heartbreaking, and transforming, and we humans are hungry for it. Reaching the ideal of forgiveness has certain requirements for patients and doctors (and sometimes sons). But kindness and forgiveness are good practice.

1

Remains

My training in unkindness began the first day of medical school.

The opening lecture of the Anatomy course took place in the oldest hospital building on campus, a coliseum-like amphitheater where bolted-down wooden desks were tiered in tight, semicircular rows. It was midmorning when I entered from the back, at the top, and the talk was already underway, the room in dusk. With the diluted projector light pushing through dust, images of body parts—eyeballs, hearts, recognizable but halved—appeared on a screen that covered the enormous wall in front of me. The lecturer, the director of the Anatomy Department, stood in the well at the bottom, a nearly vertical drop below the 120 students who were beginning four years of training. It was a lecture hall built before the age of microphones, and the acoustics were impossibly clear.

I had been warned about the severity of this instructor, about his tight Marine haircut and shoulders-back style. His voice had no modulation. It had been a humid summer and I was wearing gray shorts, but the air was chilled. I had gooseflesh. The silent room smelled of metal lubricant and floor wax. I tried to maneuver down the steep and narrow stairs to sit among my classmates; my sneakers only fit sidewise on the slick steps. The aisle seats were all taken, so I stumbled past a woman taking notes using a tiny booklight clamped to her binder and sat. I looked around, squinting, for someone I knew. Although I had missed the introduction, I knew that this first hour was to be followed by the entire class heading to the anatomy lab across the street.

The images on the screen were a lesson in realism and meant to shock. They were photographs of anatomical oddities, some exploded by disease, some still attached to bodies, others laid out on blue surgical towels: tonsillar tumors, bloodied nipples, curved spines, and split testes. Whatever Dr. Foy's background narrative—the patient's age at death, the surgical technique, the prevalence of the condition in the general population—my ears began to hum with internal white noise. I couldn't hear his words. I heard a background murmur, nothing more. My sinuses filled, my head was heavy. I tried to breathe deeply, but took in no new air; what entered was cold metal. Within a minute, I was nauseated. I attempted to shut down each of my senses. My mouth stuck together. I closed my eyes; I tried to think of the daylight outside the room. I tried to meditate. I tried to pretend I was swimming in a pond I loved. The more I felt I had to stay composed, the more I felt I couldn't.

I was twenty-two years old, and my father had been dead for almost a decade by then. I hadn't gone to the hospital on the night that he died; I'd never seen his body dead. The steady click of the projector became the metronome of his absence.

I needed to stand up. I opened my eyes and looked down into the pit of the amphitheater, forcing my vision to the lower edge of the screen as one tries to find and hold the horizon line when his boat is dipping and rolling. My classmates were sedate, silent, wide-eyed, interested. They were my age, give or take a few years, relatively recent college graduates. Like me, they were professional test-takers, rule-followers, disciplined studiers waiting for orders, Marines of the mind. Still focused on the edge of the screen, I could barely discern the outline of the person whose bass voice was narrating this introduction to the medicalized body.

"Today you will meet your first patient," Foy said.

My foot started tapping; my throat was dry. My senses were coming back and I didn't want them to. I couldn't breathe. Lifting up my folding desktop, which made a hinged snap, I stood, and the pitch of the auditorium, the altitude, gave me vertigo. My notebook slid to the floor, but I didn't bend to get it. How could I? There was no space; I was off-balance. The pages were blank anyway. I stumbled past my note-taking classmates, got to the stairs, and climbed until I was gone from the room.

The lecture hall was at the center of the original brick nineteenth-century hospital building in Manhattan. It had been the site of famously contested lectures in the history of medicine, hot arguments about theories of disease and surgical technique.

Over the decades, offices, labs, and classrooms had been built around the amphitheater, the way cooling tanks surround a nuclear core where the necessary reactions take place. Escaping the auditorium into a narrow hallway, I entered a stream of people. They looked to be patients recently released, limping and bandaged, who it seemed had given up one piece or another of themselves to one of the slides Professor Foy had projected. They looked distraught. One shook the bridge of his nose; another held her hands over her ears as if her head was banging. I stayed close to the walls, concrete as slick as the stairs of the auditorium.

Outside, the New York City street was loud, crowded, alive. The humidity made the edges of the buildings fuzzy. I tipped my head back, searching for sky between two apartment towers, sucking air until a bus coughed by. My feet were stiff. I walked down the block and found some steps to sit on. The cement left gritty imprints on my palms. I felt like a child. I had a sense that if I didn't go to the anatomy lab that day, I never would.

I waited in a shaft of sunlight for the students in my class to appear so I could join them crossing the street. I thought of the playground across from my house as a boy. My elementary school was on the far side of a hundred yards of outfield weeds and pitcher's mound and asphalt. I entered the hallowed ground through an opening in the wire fence where the dirt was rutted and the older kids had to duck to reach the field. Where were the children in this neighborhood? Where was the playground closest to this street corner?

I waited like a shamed and disqualified athlete with nowhere to go. Forty-five minutes later, blinking away the darkness of the lecture room, the students came out of the revolving door one by one, following Foy, who was moving fast, heading across the street to the lab building. I had disdain for them all; every one of them was braver than I was. A few looked at me as they passed, recognizing me from the lecture hall. No one asked me where I'd gone. I was glad for their indifference.

I joined the pack following Foy. I looked at my feet and was carried along. We moved through three doors and stood in the lab anteroom with its lockers for our books and round stub hooks for our jackets. Foy had disappeared and returned wearing a white coat, and we put on the white coats we found in our lockers for the first time. They didn't yet have our names stitched over the breast pocket—we were anonymous. If Foy remembered us at all, it wouldn't be by name.

Foy had blue eyes and sunken cheeks, and when he walked, he didn't look around; he looked straight ahead. The door to the lab was metal. It was unmarked by plaque or number. Foy opened it like a walk-in freezer. It was winter inside the room. The smell of formaldehyde was like a very high whistle, a vinegar whistle we could all now hear.

As we entered one after another, we saw dead bodies. I'd never seen a dead body before. The time I came closest was when I was thirteen, sitting in the emergency department waiting room, and my mother came to tell me that my father had died. I refused to go into the patient area to see his dead body. I couldn't bring myself to see such a confusing and monstrous thing. I had no idea what my mind or voice or body was likely to do in there with him. It had not occurred to me that he could die. He had been alive when I'd gone to sleep that night. I was afraid. Also, as long as I didn't go in to see him, he wasn't dead, some part of me imagined. Instead I sat alone in the waiting room until, twenty minutes later, my mother came back and took me home

Now, in Foy's anatomy lab, I stood clustered with my fellow students, all of us crowded together, and I heard someone say, *Let's get this over with*, and it was the first time I thought of being part of a "we." Thirty dead bodies spaced on industrial metal tables. The metal door closed behind us. From now on, we would expect death to show up in front of us. We weren't going to be surprised. I say "we" as if I knew what anyone else was expecting and would admit to.

In the breast pocket of our white coats was a rectangle of paper with a number on it. Each of the metal tables had a number, and when we found our table, we found the group of four students we'd be working with for the year. Foy stood in front of table 1. He was vain in the way he snapped on his latex gloves. We drew latex gloves from a cardboard box on the corner of each table and without vanity, slowly, carefully, watching for tiny tears, stretched them onto our fingers. We held our hands away from our bodies, as if they had to remain sterile or as a way to dissociate us from what these hands were about to do. The anatomy lab had the austerity of a machine shop. Or a professional kitchen where no one would ever bring food. Beside the silver tables were low, silver swivel stools. No table was pushed against the wall. Each was an island that groups of four or six of us could encircle to get at the body from every angle.

At first, we were like tourists watching each other rather the touring the site. We knew nothing of each other—family, religion, sense of humor, sense of violence, hungers, ethics, loves. We took our places around the tables. Did any of us want to be here? Some did, I saw, and their eagerness mystified and embarrassed me.

I expected there to be drains in the floor. I expected there to be windows that we could open to let the noxious fumes out. I expected there to be klieg lights like you'd come upon late at night on the highway, when a road crew was fixing an underpass. I expected there to be something, anything, in the room besides the gleaming silver and the gray light and the silence. I could hear the fabric of my white coat when I turned my shoulder right or left.

Our "first patients" were in clear airless plastic bags like the ones I kept clay in as a boy so that it wouldn't dry out. Their hands, feet, and skulls were wrapped in white linen. As if they'd once been huddled together and whatever had brought them to this place had worked from the edges in. Frostbite, perhaps. Or some bacteria I didn't yet know that attacked the extremities. As if they'd been horribly injured at those places that were most exposed. And now they were fully exposed except in those places.

When I was twenty-two, or twenty-three, or twenty-six, death was not urgent. It was not a pressing matter. There was no chance or practically none that I would die or that a friend would. Or that I'd see a dead body other than on TV, where it had been posed and un-deathlike, more like sleeping.

The proof that death exists left its mark. It existed thirty times over, in front of us, that morning. In that moment in the lab, I was trying to survive. Any possibility of learning had been usurped by horror. To survive, I had to control repugnance, fear, nausea. I would be expected to cut into these bodies. I wasn't sure I could do it.

My upset on the first day of medical school, I would learn later when I read the studies, was not all that unusual. Surveys reveal that approximately 5 percent of medical students have a severe immediate physical reaction to their first day in the anatomy lab. I was part of this exclusive 5 percent who experienced a "strong negative arousal." These studies do not provide data as to what pitiful percentage has a strong negative arousal *before* they've even gotten to the lab. Only a fraction of this 5 percent reports a "persistent and serious disturbance." Presumably, among the 5 percent are those who run away, never to become doctors, but the authors don't enumerate or comment on this group.

Consistently across the many studies of first-year medical students, more than 50 percent report some "reaction"—a drop in concentration, for example—to beginning Anatomy. Is it possible that the other 50 percent truly have no reaction, or is this survey response the deliberate refusal to admit to an emotional response, the beginning of what will become a deeply ingrained habit of simply proceeding? International studies reveal that American medical students find the anatomy room more stressful than those in Europe do. Why? Are European students more likely to have been to a wake? Are American students oversensitive? Are Americans shielded from death in almost every context? Are the British and Irish psychologically more resilient? Or are Americans more willing to report psychological distress? In these studies, the great majority of medical students note that the dissecting room is a relatively unimportant cause of stress compared to the amount of work and exam anxiety.

In academic journals, some authors advise about anatomy lab: "Caution must be exercised to ensure that students do not concentrate on affective factors at the expense of learning." Others suggest: "Dissection is primarily an occasion for studying anatomy, which can be disrupted if attention is focused unduly on death and dying."

Students who continue past the first day of lab are extremely unlikely to drop out of medical school, nearly universally graduating on time. Indeed, most students report that they feel mentally prepared for dissection. Particularly those who have seen a dead body before—which I hadn't.

The detachment that some suggest enables one to practice medicine begins in the anatomy lab: the jokes, the laughing that signifies toughness, the gallows humor. (Foy wouldn't have been amused—he'd heard it all—but he wouldn't have minded any of it either; he understood the mechanics of camaraderie, although there was none of it when he was around.) The lapses of taste help to escape the tyranny of the serious.

Participating in anatomy lab presents what psychologists call the "white bear challenge." Here's the test: starting now, can you not think about a white bear for the next minute now that I've asked you not to think of a white bear? Of course you can't. This failure is what psychologist Daniel Wegner calls theory of ironic process. By issuing the challenge, you demonstrate the futility of the struggle. Maybe we win for a while by using what Wegner calls metacognition, our ability to think about, and therefore control, what we're thinking about. One can force alternative thoughts into the mind for a while, but the white bear challenge is almost impossible to win for long. Still, metacognition is a medical student's most useful skill, this pushing away of the image of a white bear, or anxiety. It is perhaps the great skill of the surgeon.

The internal mechanism for sabotaging our effort at suppressing white bear thoughts is also potent. Metacognition is a self-monitoring process, but it often goes wrong—the studies show that when we are tired, stressed, attempting to multitask, suffering from the mental load doctors walk around with, the monitoring process itself starts to occupy the cognitive stage, and suddenly all you will be able to think about is white bears. Not wanting to think certain thoughts, not wanting to feel certain emotions isn't enough to eliminate them. This failure is what happened to me in that vertiginous lecture hall. I didn't want to think about being a doctor; I didn't want to think about my father, dead. But these are the things I thought about.

At its best, metacognition enables us to recognize when we are being unreasonable, or being affected by our own distress, and then we can do something about it.

"While there is clearly a need for medical schools to address such issues as mortality, it is questionable whether this should be a formal aspect of the Anatomy course," the educators write. Nearly every medical student requests that education about death be either available or compulsory in the preclinical years, perhaps running concurrently with Anatomy. Death Ed is the name of this imaginary medical school course I never took. Death Education has indeed been added to the medical curriculum at some institutions as an introduction to grief, as a booster for metacognitive skills, and as a professional school's good ethical measure, with the hope that such courses might mitigate the overly confident overtreatment of dying patients that will occur years later by many physicians, and assuage the consequent psychological discomfort and lack of self-confidence these physicians have facing families after the death of a patient.

Driver's Ed courses are not entirely effective. There are still plenty of accidents and bad drivers. "Keep your eyes on the middle line and both hands on the wheel," my best friend's girlfriend said when she was teaching me to drive in her VW. My father didn't teach me to drive. By the time I was ready for my learner's permit, he was dead. So how much would Death Ed help? "Medical students' empathy tends to wane with each year of education, and by their third year many medical students want to distance themselves from their patients." So conclude the authors of one of the largest studies following new students from matriculation to graduation. In fact, most of the waning occurs in the first year, during Anatomy.

Medical students learn a thousand new words during the first year of medical school, and many are anatomical, Latinate and beautiful. In the lab we said "cadaver," not "corpse." "Corpse" is a heavy word, waterlogged, a body that needs to be disposed of. A corpse belongs in a mass grave. A cadaver is something else. A cadaver has been kept, placed aside as part of a ritual: abra-cadaver. A corpse is a war body and comes with a hint of trauma. A corpse has been stranded, sunken, lost interest in, slaughtered with a grievance. A cadaver has been prepared after dying. It's been shaved, shaped, cleaned, wrapped. A corpse is pitiful; a cadaver has a value. It's like the difference between a victim and a martyr.

The politically correct term is "donor." Those medical educators who use the word "donor" are the same ones who claim that anatomy lab is the first site of patient care, that the donor is the student's first patient and first professional responsibility, that there is a direct line to later clinical work. I once heard Foy also refer to a body as a "cadaveric specimen." "Donor" is preferable, some authors write, because "cadaver" is too impersonal. "Donor" emphasizes the gifting aspect, the contribution to science, and suggests an element of trust. The donor trusted that we would make good use of his or her body, the remains. The donor is the teacher who will guide our training. Why did I object to Foy calling her "my first patient"? Because my cadaver was not suffering (as far as I knew), could not be cured, would be disassembled without being made whole again.

When we are children, we have our first experiences in and expectations of the way others express suffering. As we grow older, we come to empathize with people by conceiving of and imagining a person in pain, by the way we come to see suffering expressed, by the way that a person in pain treats us. Yet as a student of medicine, the first person I was offered the chance to empathize with was dead. This set a certain tone. Because we can't empathize with the dead; they are past pain and suffering. I say "we" because, looking back, it's a way to protest the culture of isolation that developed at that moment and that remains the culture of doctors.

Historically and currently, anatomy is the entrance to medicine. It is the first striving for a professional ethic of stoicism based on the formula "emotion equals weakness equals lack of scientific objectivity." It is the opening test of emotional competence. It is the demonstration that you are no longer like your friends who have entered other lines of work or study. It is the time when students first fear that the mind's mastery over the heart is tentative and may not hold.

Perhaps I should have taken my disturbance as the first, but not the last, sign of my unsuitability for the profession.

Anatomy lab is about not letting yourself and others know how difficult this experience is, how time spent with a cadaver affects you. As the white bear challenge teaches, we do not have perfect self-control. Not wanting to think about death, not wanting to feel certain emotions isn't sufficient to eliminate them. Yet for the rest of our days as doctors we are meant to have such control: we will not share our distress.

The creation myth of the profession holds that cold detachment creates the conditions for, in fact consolidates, the purely technical competence the future physician will need in order to deal with the anxieties inherent in his or her work.

Merriam-Webster's defines "detached" as "not involved by emotion."

The detachment is often first recognized only months or years later when a friend or family member becomes ill. You begin asking questions, very detailed, very careful. You know too much. You've seen too much, and this prevents you from being as emotionally helpful as you might have been otherwise. You are now the doctor; your uncle is now the patient. Patients are not friends. You focus on the symptoms as a phenomenon, not something that happens to you, your mother or uncle. Your uncle is dying, and you listen not as a nephew but as a professional deciding whether to second-guess, whether to offer advice and treatment options, whether to be honest that any reassurance is hollow. You practice a kind of double-entry emotional bookkeeping, enmeshed in a family illness while keeping the distance of a medical perspective.

Rather than disclosing too much about myself—my judgments and contempt, my moods and fear—I am expected to keep my distance from patients. This is what doctors call composure, and it is a form of self-protection. I learned this composure on the first day of anatomy lab, the first day of medical school, when I refused to let anyone know that I was either impressed or upset. Admit to nothing. Not a feeling, not a doubt. But isn't this true of all students who are trying to elude discovery, disguising weaknesses in order to seem stronger or better than they are? Isn't this true of many doctors, who still deny that distancing is a choice?

I was thirteen when my father died. The career plans of thirteen-year-old suburban American boys are banal: drummer, professional athlete, doctor, professional sports team's doctor. I read biographies of heroes and *Rolling Stone* magazine. I read on my back on the floor, arms extended upward, so if I fell asleep, the pages would fall on my face and wake me. I still played on the floor, board games, games with dice and math and small metal balls, and teams that won and lost. Do you know any thirteen-year-old boys? When they speak at all, they admit to nothing. Not a feeling, not a doubt. They never think about the future. These characteristics make them perfect soldiers in certain cultures. These characteristics, if they persist for another decade, make them perfect medical students; and, if they persist for a decade more, make them unkind doctors.

I understood later why Foy had covered the hands; he was sparing us, although he didn't seem the type. Unwrapped, the stiffened hands would look menacing and inhuman. I understood why he had covered the feet. Nail polish would be *too* human: chipped, flaky, the undercolor of a church fresco from another century. I understood why he had wrapped the heads in their own bags, with cords tied around the neck. So that none of us recognized someone we might have known. It seemed possible that my father was somewhere in this room.

The only way I could remain in the room (Foy called it a "lab," but what was the experiment?), and not run away as I had earlier from the images on the lecture hall screen, was to become an actor. I would project nonchalance and comfort. I would be an actor portraying a strangely limited character, one whose private range of public emotions—frustration, irony, disgust—had narrowed. When I walked offstage and took off my white coat, when I returned to T-shirt and shorts, would my fuller set of emotions return? Could I be vulnerable in one part of my life and not in another? Every time I put on a white coat, would I be limited in these ways again? Was that the role of a doctor?

I looked at and then away from our "first patients." This looking away was instinctual. In part it was cowardice, but also we are instinctively opposed to abandonment, and abandonment is what we sense when we first look at the dead. There was a granular intensity to the shadowless light in the room, every surface vivid and distinct. As in prayer, there was an obliterative quiet that opened up space in my thoughts.

Close up, I could see that the metal tables had scalpel scratches. The scalpels came out of individual aluminum packets that we ripped open at the top like wilderness meals. I was afraid that I would be the one asked to lift our body from its clear bag, and if so, why would the others around my table trust someone who ran out of the first class to do anything? But I could see that they didn't trust themselves either. But some had, somehow, at some time during their lives, learned to work automatically.

We didn't need to lift the body from the bag. We could unzip it and fold it down, working with the cadaver still in the bag on the table. I kept up the internal monologue about my father I had begun earlier—I must have gone to the funeral, why I couldn't remember; maybe there wasn't a funeral?—trying to keep the undiscussed and the unmentioned from overtaking me. The role was becoming clearer: I was an actor who would say nothing aloud.

A woman: I was relieved ours was a woman. She was a human body, but there was no human presence. She was dark and cool, like doubt.

That left twenty-nine others I would have to check to see if my father was among us.

We cut on this first day. There was no such thing as innocent bystanding. I held a blade like any executioner, firmly, to calm the shaking. We cut slowly. There was nothing abrupt. We weren't in a hurry. This class would go on for hours, for months. We were more afraid that we were able to do it than not able.

The flesh was hide drained of color, the muscle stringy, dense as beef jerky, but with an odor between turpentine and shoe polish that brought the tip of my tongue to the roof of my mouth, trying to wipe it away. We sprayed from small bottles (water, propylene glycol, ethyl alcohol, and fabric softener) to prevent desiccation. In our white coats, we were unsentimental butchers inhaling embalming stink. There was no spilling fluid, no serum, mucus, or blood. There were no time constraints. Embalmed, the cadavers could sit at room temperature for years without decomposition.

Dissection of the head would come last, months away. The mystery of who lay beneath the wrapping: I was relieved to wait. But the first day I also felt I wanted unveiling to come sooner. I thought of finding bravery, of going into the lab alone at night, lighting votive candles and unwinding the linen from the other twenty-nine cadavers' faces until I found him. I could see my father again and get past it, get on to my medical career and the rest of my life.

<hr>

Perhaps anatomy lab should not be the entrance to medicine. If we have no reason to be kind to our "patient," will we necessarily be kind to the ones who come after?

Weeks passed. Our tests involved moving from body to body, a single part tagged on each. Examinations as examinations. What artery is this? What foramen is this? What nerve is this? A challenge of memory, sweat trickling down my back. Motionless bodies lack purpose. The body's purpose, I understood, in this course and forevermore as a doctor, was to serve as a test. Cadaver training made the body into a map to memorize in hyperdetail, along with the physiology. It turned the inevitability of death into facts, into science, map point to map point with a great sense of mission. There was a great satisfaction in getting the landmarks right.

Which is to say nothing of the awe. The excitement of discovery and the privileged, incredible, touchable view, the human layers. There was the forbidden, viscous marvel of structural beauty, the original form as function. I experienced both shock and comprehension at the miniature valves, the air sacs, the marrow—surprise at things that make perfect physical sense. We took the body apart, in parts: thorax, upper extremities, lower extremities, neck. We left the head wrapped. I was next in a line of anatomists going back centuries. Working from clues and hints—clues to chaos, hints of tragedy—working at secret holes and cul-de-sacs. I felt alive and sinning.

I would come to know something of the maps of the twenty-nine others in the lab—not as intimately as our own cadaver, but I would know aspects of each. The truth is, I can't remember what my cadaver looked like. I spent every day with her for nine months, taking her apart piece by piece, and I couldn't pick her out of a cadaver lineup. If Foy had moved the tables around, I wouldn't have been able to find her. Death steals individuality, steals color and breath and expression and the volume of cells.

Would I remember his body? I had known it only as a boy knows his father, with the memory of eyes fixed on visible sources of power—shoulders and hands and gestures, and facial language, his frown of disappointment. He had been dead a long time.

Weeks passed. One student dreamed of cadavers floating by while she stood in chest-high water, another of carrying a bloodied bone in a coffee can. One dreamed of the inside of her own heart. In the bath, she could see through his skin to her internal organs. Another, at the supermarket, reached for an item and saw his hand as a cadaver's. He imagined that the cancer metastases he'd found in the lungs of his cadaver could spread to the cadavers nearby. She dreamed that her head and neck had been removed and she could see down inside her body. He dreamed the men moving the furniture into his new apartment were wearing masks made of the same materials as the gloves in the lab.

She dreamed the cadaver had the face of a boyfriend from years before. He became disgusted by grease and was unable to cut into the chicken thigh he was served at dinner.

With their knives, my classmates were illogically gentle. I wanted to be violent. I wanted to use force. I wanted to puncture the wet and resistant skin a thousand times until my blade was dull. I wanted the free pass that came from admitting what we were doing. Pity my cadaver? Irrelevant. She wasn't my patient; she was dead. I was angry that there was nothing I could do for her and so, paradoxically, I wanted to harm this body I couldn't harm. She wouldn't flinch or wince or pull away. She wasn't going anywhere. I wanted to be careless and jagged and imprecise as I would never be if she were alive.

There was no reason to be disrespectful to a cadaver. But I did not feel unkind. What seems like mutilation foretells the future doctor's forceful procedures during the brutality of surgeries, I told myself. Here, as there, muscles would be ripped, ribs separated, intestines laid on a table and then stuffed back. Here, as there, I would take her body apart, cut pieces away, and put them in buckets.

Weeks passed. Her knees bent stiffly. Her hips rotated against contraction. We swept away fascia and plunged fingers in. We partitioned and understood, committed to memory. If each of us were alone, it would have been different, but because we were in a group these actions did not feel depraved. We talked little because we didn't want to disturb each other. We didn't ask, What does it mean to be dead, to have this happen to you?

When her bone snapped, it sounded like the collapse of a chair. I wondered about future patients I might harm.

Doctors have rates of suicide twice as high as the general population, and higher than other professions. Each year, it would take the equivalent of a class around those tables to replace the number of doctors who kill themselves. Medical students enter school with mental health profiles similar to their peers. Twenty-five percent develop depression before they graduate; 10 percent have thoughts of killing themselves. Where does the list of experiences that lead to an increased risk suicide begin?

Doctors almost never leave their bodies to anatomy labs.

I daydreamed: If we dumped the buckets on the street outside, would the city animals eat the flesh? Alms for the pigeons. This would not be how I would think of surgical patients, I told myself. But this first time, it was not dissection as much as destruction. And my cadaver was *not* my patient. I did this work for my interest, not hers. Embalmed, silent, motionless, cadavers are not people. They were. Or they are, and they were.

Should I have been ashamed that I was not disgusted by these thoughts? After all, I'd been given a gift. I was moving toward a career. I should have been grateful and reverent. I should have celebrated and commemorated. It wasn't appropriate. But what was appropriate?

I needed a father to rage against when I was thirteen. I hadn't had one. Now I was twenty-three. Now I was thirteen.

If he wasn't one of the thirty in the room, if I'd never seen him dead, if I didn't know where he was buried, it raised the possibility that he hadn't been buried at all. He had not left his body to science as far as I knew. I must have gone to the funeral, but I couldn't remember. I would have admitted to the emotional weakness of running away from the first lecture of medical school before I'd have admitted to that. Our cadavers' heads remained wrapped.

There was a waiting list to get into an Ivy League medical school as a cadaver—the last chance to reach a lifelong goal. Did Foy have a list of the cadavers' names? Did he run a cross-match against the last names of the students in his class? That wouldn't really protect one of us from coming across an aunt, a former teacher, a neighbor. What were the odds?

I could be wrong about moving the Anatomy course to later in the medical curriculum. Perhaps the current order is the correct sequence of classes. The capacity to hold and balance the emotional and intellectual aspects of the work, to accept and manage the tension between them, is the enduring conflict for doctors. Since Anatomy anticipated this central issue of a medical career, why not raise it on the first day? Sooner or later we must be taught not to reveal too much or feel too much. When we meet patients we will not blush at nakedness, or cry when hurting them.

The curricular question is: Sooner or later? Sooner: Anatomy brings out our worst—disgust, frustration, self-loathing—and the best way to explore these emotions that we will later hide is by our work with the dead. Showing us the end of life first will make us pay more attention to life. Later: it's better to first learn how to worry about someone other than ourselves, a real patient, because when we are with the dead, we are only thinking of ourselves.

Later we would be taught to be managers of patients' complex biology and the technology needed to maintain it. We would be trained as problem solvers under the paradigm that all problems are soluble, that death was a mark of failure. Yet on the table in the lab was an insoluble problem.

If one believes that dissection represents the student's first encounter with a "patient," then it might be reasonable to predict that the coping mechanisms the student employs will be ones she or he uses when confronted with living patients. But there is no evidence that the difficulty or ease of the actions we perform on cadavers help us prepare for agonizing moments in the lives of patients. If walking into a room of cadavers teaches us anything, it's that we do not know how to prepare for being overwhelmed in advance.

Weeks passed. For many, the dreams continued. The taboo dreams of skinning people, the murderer's dreams of decapitation, the criminal's dreams of hemisection, of carcasses hanging like cows in freezers, would visit us. Death terror. After the body had been taken apart, literally, piece by piece, limb from limb, in those last weeks, when we uncovered the face, we would know who we'd done this to.

I knew nothing about her. I didn't know when she died or what year she was born or any of the dateless minutes in between. I knew nothing about her life—not her schooling, or talents, or friends, or children, not her good luck or bad, if she prayed when she fell ill or was stoic, without metaphysical complaint. I knew only that she died.

There were several ways to pass an Anatomy course. For me, it was a matter not only of learning the pathways of nerves and the routes of veins but also of learning that every time I would see a dead body, it would still be all right to stop acting, to let sadness wash over me.

I was thinking of him—that is, what remained of my few memories of him—without wanting to, week after week. My white bear.

There is a psychoanalytic hypothesis that many students enter medicine because of their own fear of death, and that by entering a profession where death and dying are frequent, they hope to conquer the fear, and at the same time conquer death. I came to medical school thinking about my life and the lives of my future patients, but without understanding that the dissection of a cadaver is the first in a long series of encounters with death. Still, the idea of death, the fear of it, ghosted me. In the lab, I never entertained the thought that this cadaver would eventually be me. I did not imagine myself dead. Unlike many of my classmates, I was at least spared this. I was too busy imagining him there.

What remained of him for me was not alive, but it was not dead either.

Years later we would be omnipotent. It was the beginning of The Deal. Doctors would be steady and professional, illness would be managed, and things would go well. We would be defiant, concede little to illness. The illness we loathed. If all behaved as if nothing was very wrong, nothing would go wrong and everyone would be thankful, saved. From the first days, we were inclined, even taught, to shut down our expressions, some of our feelings. We smiled with our mouths closed.

To be an optimist you must be in denial about lots of things.

Maybe there wasn't a funeral. Maybe there was no burial. I'd never asked my mother. Perhaps he was alive and there was still a way for me to save him, I'd fantasized that first day in the auditorium when Foy projected his images.

My panic, the first day, was about loss. In the past I had mourned my father's absence, but never before his being dead, a cadaver, a corpse.

2

Losing Control

Every doctor enters an unspoken contract with his or her patients, according to which the doctor is expected to be endlessly patient. Doctors make an implicit pledge always to retain their self-control, because if they let it run out, frustration shows and unkindness erupts. Sometimes this contract gets breached.

Beatriz always smelled of cherries and had a slow, coy smile. By the time I saw her that August, on an afternoon when the summer sun coming through the window at the far end of my exam room made me feel bad for the withered plant on the sill and for the fact that I still hadn't bought curtains, I had been caring for her for three years, since her daughter Dahlia was four. By then I was forty-five, and for over twenty years I had cared for thousands of HIV patients like Beatriz because I had chosen to make HIV disease the focus of my career. I had seen, close-up, the greatest medical achievement of my generation—the conversion of a fatal disease into a chronic one. I had watched the life expectancy of a person with HIV who faithfully took his or her daily medication grow until it had become approximately the same as that of person without HIV. I had seen, too, that without medication, or without the correct use of medication, all survival bets were off. Beatriz's medication use had been erratic, and for three years I had been patient with her about this. The restraint that had enabled me to override my instinctual response to her self-destructive behavior was gone.

I hadn't given Beatriz the results of her HIV test, but I was the first doctor she saw after learning the diagnosis. I remember, at our first visit, how slowly she moved. Although she was only thirty-seven, it was as if she lacked adrenaline. I couldn't imagine her running, or even moving fast. She seemed to collapse into the thin metal chair in my office; her neck naturally tipped her chin to her chest, and she spoke softly, looking at the floor.

Her daughter Dahlia came to this first visit of Beatriz's and brought Barbie dolls with her. She sat them on her chair, and kneeled on the dirty linoleum floor in front of them, silently mouthing advice and instruction, her back to the examining table where her mother sat on the white butcher-shop paper. She had her mother's soft brown eyes.

I asked Beatriz who knew about her test results. No one except her husband, she said, the only man she'd been with, the one who had infected her with HIV and sometimes lived with her, a guy with long, stringy hair and sharp teeth I'd seen in the waiting area, reading a magazine standing up. She wanted to keep it that way. She hadn't told her sister who lived in town. She hadn't told her mother, a thousand miles away in the Dominican hills of Cibao, who was dealing with her own diabetes. She hadn't told her best friend, who'd been urging her to leave her husband for years anyway. If anyone found out about her HIV, there would be humiliation, guilt, embarrassment; there was the risk of their fear, blame, the unkind words, the possibility of withdrawal, and a refusal and unwillingness to help. While she might find some support, she didn't expect any. Beatriz turned down my suggestion to speak to a counselor, as this would mean the revelation of her secret to another person, and I was concerned about her isolation.

I found myself speaking in code at that first visit, not using the acronym "HIV" in front of Dahlia, who at four wouldn't have understood if I had. Beatriz and I never used the acronym in the office in front of Dahlia. It became part of the contract between us.

There are enigmatic illnesses whose prognoses are uncertain, in which well-being comes and goes unpredictably; they are medical stories with unfathomable plots. Where the story is variable, I share with my patient every conceivable possibility; I am soft in my approach because, for the patient, not knowing what will happen and what to expect is a kind of pain itself. And then there are illnesses with predictable paths and trajectories, and I can talk about upcoming events and confidently offer my experience.

I am harder-voiced, less tolerant: my sympathy depends on the patient's willingness to follow my recommendation, because here the illness is controllable, and I want the patient to be as well, for her own good. HIV was this form of illness.

My recommendation to Beatriz early on was to start treatment. Using our code, we called them "pills," not "HIV medications," not "medicines to prevent the progression to AIDS," and by our third visit Beatriz had agreed to begin.

I saw her every three months to monitor lab work, which indicated whether her virus was under control, and to see how she was doing. Beatriz was a small woman who carried an enormous canvas shoulder bag that held a sweater—she was always cold—and a book for her daughter, snacks and tubes of skin lotion, keys, bracelets, and Kleenex. Dahlia still came to every appointment with her Barbies. She found new places in the room for her dolls to visit. Sometimes she sat them on the large slate windowsill that looked out over the city, if it wasn't too hot, or she disappeared into the corner behind the exam table. Sometimes she carried them to the small metal sink, pulled over the chair to stand on, and washed their hair.

Beatriz and Dahlia were obviously close, but they never interacted much in the office. From the first visit, there seemed to be an understanding that this was Mama's time, not to be interrupted. Dahlia never asked me or her mother a question. She always pranced into the room in front of her mother—of course Beatriz moved slowly, heavily—as if it were *her* appointment, and then she disappeared into her silent play. Even at seven, that August afternoon, she was silent as a cat. Beatriz and I sometimes spoke in Spanish, which was easier for her than English, and she got to correct my mistakes. But she liked to practice her English, which she believed she should have spoken better given that she'd lived in the United States for more than a decade. Dahlia spoke both languages perfectly and looked up at me when I mispronounced or misconjugated, and then, teacher's helper, looked over at her mother, who was already *tsk*-ing me into improvement, her one sign of liveliness. Seemingly absorbed in play, the child missed nothing and was alert to everything.

From the first month after beginning anti-HIV therapy, Beatriz admitted to missing doses. When I tried to understand why, she yawned to make clear that her life was tiring and every dose was an effort, and that my questions, after a certain point, tired her. She claimed that she understood the importance of taking the pills correctly, although she didn't promise to do better. Patients tell me that my eyes almost never betray any emotion except disappointment. Beatriz must have known that I was disappointed.

Beatriz's admission that she was missing pills, present from almost the start, was reasserted every three months. "I forget. I don't keep them with me," she said. I warned her at every visit that forgetting to take her pills two or three days a week would get her in trouble, that her condition would only be held in check by close adherence to a pill schedule. I told her that her body needed a constant, regular level of medication, water on a fire, to keep the problem under control. I told her how her disease gained power when she missed doses. How the disease would grow stronger and the medication would lose its potency and we would run out of options for new ones. Her good health depended on control of the problem, which depended on this medication adherence.

Beatriz had a special kind of sadness, asking for little, and thanking me for nothing. Every three months she returned to report the same difficulty with her pills and I would sit on my rolling chair and try to get a sense of why she wasn't fully adherent and why she kept coming back if only to tell me the same thing. But I looked forward to seeing how Dahlia had grown, and Beatriz's passivity usually kept me attentive; I kept trying to come up with new memory devices to improve her pill-taking, hoping that it was simple forgetfulness.

On one visit, she had accepted a pillbox from me. At the next, when she admitted that she forgot to fill it, I preloaded twelve pillboxes in my office, one for each week until our next meeting. She was still missing doses by the following visit, so we discussed ritualizing the event, putting the pillbox or pill bottles next to her toothbrush, where she was sure to go twice a day. She rarely left the house. She cleaned, she sewed her daughter's dresses, and she cooked the standard Dominican starch and fried food diet that could slow anyone for two hours after a meal. Could she take her pills with *desayuno y cena*? She had tried to set an alarm to remember her evening dose.

I thought of engaging her husband. He nodded at me from across the room whenever I escorted her out to the waiting area. He was a part-time mechanic and sold prescription pills to addicts for his real income. He took Beatriz's arm when they walked to the elevator. Dahlia held his hand and tried to skip, tried to tug the two of them along. He was clearly involved with his family, but Beatriz didn't want to ask for his help when I suggested it. She smiled her pained smile as if there was nothing she could do to help me, or herself.

We had established a lousy pattern: I would scold, and Beatriz would shrug or monosyllabically rationalize missing her pills; I was never sure what she was thinking. When she arrived in August, there was evidence from her blood work three months before, and from her February report three months earlier, that she was missing enough doses that her virus was now dangerously out of control. I was exasperated with Beatriz. Getting her to change her behavior seemed hopeless and no longer worth my effort to try to help. This thought made me feel incompetent and empty and defeated.

I counted on a professional life of self-control; all doctors do. After all, aren't doctors always overriding hardwired responses like fear, like disgust with the sights and smells of a clinical schedule, in order to get through the day?

There are three ways of thinking about self-control. One model views it as a skill. As with any learned skill, self-control remains roughly constant when applied over time, for instance across an afternoon of seeing patients where I keep my worst thoughts silent and do not blurt out something that could be hurtful or insulting. A second model envisions self-control as a brain system that remains in standby mode until it is pressed into action. Once activated (for instance, when I first step into my office and am primed by the first patient of the day), the system of good and controlled behavior remains in operation for a time, making further acts of self-control easier. A third model imagines that self-control resembles energy. In this view, an act of self-control (with a patient, or even in a nonmedical domain, such as an argument with my son before work) involves a kind of exertion that expends energy and thereby depletes the supply available for the next experience. Unless the supply is very large, initial acts of self-regulation should deplete it, impairing subsequent self-control. In this third model, adapting to any stress may involve a "psychic cost," and one stress makes the next one more likely. In all three models, self-control is unconscious, performing its function automatically.

Researchers have tested which of the three models applies by asking volunteers to engage in an initial self-controlling activity and then testing their self-control during a subsequent activity. For instance, one group of volunteers is asked to watch a funny movie clip. The experimenter tells the participants that they will be videotaped while watching the film and it is thus essential to try to conceal and suppress any emotional reaction (an act of self-control). Meanwhile, a second group of volunteers is instructed to let their emotions flow while watching the clip, without any attempt to hide or deny these feelings, no self-control required. Both groups watch ten minutes from a Robin Williams movie. (The same experiment has been done with a sad clip from *Terms of Endearment*.)

After the movie, the same volunteers are asked to help the experimenter collect some preliminary data for "future research," a ruse to conceal the purpose of the second self-control task. This task is an anagram game, unscrambling sets of letters. The anagrams require effort; success requires some degree of self-control, dealing with the frustration of the difficult game. Assuming that before the experiment both groups would have, on average, a roughly equal ability to do anagrams, the three models of self-control would have different predictions about anagram performance after the movie. The energy model (#3) would predict the volunteers who controlled themselves during the movie would have poorer anagram performance than the others because their self-control would be depleted; they wouldn't try as hard or concentrate as well, their focus exhausted.

In this experiment, the researchers found that the group that was asked to control their emotions during the Robin Williams clip performed less well at the subsequent self-control task than the group that had been allowed to react freely. Similar results—confirming the "psychic cost" model—have been reported in dozens of similar experiments. Restraint, it seems, is based on some limited capacity such that engaging self-control quickly consumes it, leaving one in a depleted state. Some valuable resource of the self is depleted by an initial act of volition and discipline; further attempts of self-control are prone to failure. How long this exhausted state lasts and how long until one's energy recovers is highly individual and uncertain.

That August day, Beatriz came for a regular visit. Dahlia accompanied her, as usual; she wore flowered shorts. She'd taken out her Barbies and disappeared into their world like any other day, moving them from hiding place to hiding place. I was sitting on my rolling seat, sweating. I could see that the convertibles on the highway had their tops down, and the sun's glare made me squint at Beatriz, who reported she'd had diarrhea for a month, the predictable, inevitable story of uncontrolled HIV.

"I have to go to the bathroom too much," she said. "I do not want to go out because I am afraid I will need a bathroom too fast." She sniffed; she was humiliated. She wouldn't look up from her blue espadrilles. She kept her hands over her abdomen. She rarely complained; I knew her symptoms were really bothering her. I'd gotten her latest blood test results back. They were getting worse and I was upset.

She was sitting on the white paper of the examining table when I asked, loudly, "Are you daring your HIV to kill you?" Her legs made a sharp movement and she was suddenly standing. I could see the sweat tracks her thighs had left on the paper. I had never seen her move quickly. Her head swiveled, checked the corners of the room. Where was Dahlia?

Beatriz looked at me with panic and disappointment. I had disappointed her. She had asked me for exactly one thing in three years: never say "HIV" or "AIDS" in front of Dahlia. And that's exactly what I'd done.

Dahlia came out from the small space behind the examining table. Her eyes were filled with tears. She'd heard me say "HIV." She was seven, but she knew about HIV. She knew her mother would die.

I'd said three letters and I had irreparably changed the relationship of mother and daughter. Embarrassment and regret, like a heavy hot towel slapped down on my face, reddened my jaw and cheeks. I had violated the contract of self-control with Beatriz, and in a second violation I had certainly altered her bond with Dahlia.

Beatriz grabbed her shoulder bag, told her daughter to get her things, took Dahlia's hand, and pulled her out the door.

I saw the patient scheduled after Beatriz, and the one after that, and the one after that, as if continuing to do my job and completing some evaluable quantity of visits erased my mistake. My throat ached. My head was a globe of screaming nerves. Why hadn't I been able to restrain myself that day with Beatriz? I have been thinking about her and trying to understand my capacity for self-control ever since.

At every other visit I had been able to resist the impulse to be brutally honest with Beatriz. I had never expressed my anger about her lousy pill-taking or told her not to come back until she took better care of herself. I had never said things that would have been easy to say because I knew it would carry a long-term cost and violate the rules and guidelines of the contract I made with patients. This day, I hadn't been paying attention. I'd forgotten Dahlia was in the room, but as I went over it all again, I knew that was not an adequate explanation. It suggested that I was generally inattentive, or distracted, or suffered occasionally from memory lapses. I was letting myself off too easily.

So does the depletion model explain what happened to me with Beatriz on that August day? If self-control always has limits, had I been depleted by a patient whom I'd seen before Beatriz's appointment? Was I unable to override the natural impulse to shock her into pill adherence because my self-regulating strength had deteriorated? I would like to say that I was exhausted that day from a long night on call. I would like to attribute my loss of control with Beatriz to the hard work of caring for a difficult patient who'd come in earlier that day, or a fight with my wife on the phone, or an argument with a staff member in the hall over missing supplies in the hour before Beatriz arrived. But I couldn't think of anyone or anything to blame but myself.

But I do remember feeling a kind of depletion when I saw her that day. Or rather, I felt fatigue, boredom, disappointment, and anger, the emotions of depletion. But what, or who, had depleted me then? There was no other person, event, or activity that had sapped my control. It was Beatriz, who was now symptomatic from her HIV after three years of taking her medication incorrectly: Beatriz had exhausted me. I had a kind of Beatriz fatigue.

To return to the depletion model of self-control, let me suggest a modified version. Engaging in self-control at Time 1 with Beatriz—and here Time 1 was my previous visit with her, a visit so filled with annoyance and impatience with her nonadherence that even though it was three months earlier it was fresh in my mind and felt like an hour before—led me to less restraint at Time 2 (this hour in August), although I don't believe that I was depleted. Rather, at the August visit my *motivation* had shifted. My usual "ought-to" goal (be nice) changed to a "have-to" goal (be honest—that is, be angry), and the expression of my "have-to" goal was to be confrontational, to yell and be careless. It felt meaningful and right to accuse her of poor self-care in the service of creating the possibility of a greater reward: Beatriz would finally change. I had to try. I hadn't really *lost* control. I had *less* control than I'd had at past visits with her, but I still had some control; I had, after all, calmly taken a history of her symptoms. It wasn't that I *couldn't* control myself, it was that I didn't *want to* control myself. My relative depletion (from her admitted non-adherence at every visit before) stoked my desire to be harsh because I wanted to be harsh that August day. That's what I believe today.

It was strangely gratifying to lose control in August. I yelled suddenly, unexpectedly, easily. My yelling was not a matter of inattention or distraction. It was enjoyable; it felt good; I must have told myself it was for *her* good. Yelling, unfortunately, disastrously, included the word "HIV," which I had promised never to say.

When we say that to become a doctor is to join a respected profession, we mean that doctors, during their workday in the hospital or office, are assured authority. By completing medical school, they have put themselves in a position where authority— knowing how the body works, having the ability to fix it—over another person, his patient, is, for better or worse, guaranteed. This is a profession where the doctor is the one, after all, who is *expected* to know, whom patients seek out to gain knowledge they want and need. Doctors have perhaps been drawn to the profession for the security of authority, although publicly we tell the story of helping or caring, which may be true as well, and complementary. This authority (limited in place and time to office hours) is never meant to be threatening—its purpose is teaching and treatment and relief, the benefits of knowledge and experience—but it does create a distance between doctor and patient. This distance must be bearable, and even useful, for both the patient, who must feel able to say anything, and the doctor, who must exhibit self-control for a greater purpose. Any sense of authority can be undermined, most notably when expert advice is neglected or ignored. When it was undermined, in my case, by Beatriz's nonadherence, I needed to control myself, and I didn't.

So perhaps there's still another version of what happened that day. Maybe what had been depleted was my sense of purpose. Maybe I didn't want to accept that Beatriz wouldn't listen to me. She'd come to me for my experience and expertise, and then she'd gone ahead and made her own decisions for three years. She'd taken up my time, and I expected some acceptance of my advice in return. As each three-month visit approached, I would think again about why she was noncompliant, and what it was that she really wanted from life. The reasons for missing pills almost didn't matter. There was shame about her illness, true forgetfulness, fatalism, magical thinking that missing pills meant she didn't really have HIV, an inability to find the inner resources, the self-control, necessary to take pills for the rest of her life. There were a million possible reasons.

Did I really forget that Dahlia was there? I still ask myself. Was that possible, even if she was invisible, out of sight with her Barbies behind the examination table? Or did I unconsciously mean to use to Beatriz's daughter against her? Did I unconsciously want Dahlia to pop up and ask her mother to do better, to live longer?

Would it have been any better if I had yelled what I had when her daughter wasn't present, if I'd sent her daughter from the room beforehand? Was my trespass worse because Dahlia was present, because I was forcing Beatriz to face her selfishness and look at her daughter?

Anger is a judgment. Did I have a right to judge Beatriz? A doctor's kindness means more than bearing a patient's vulnerability, sharing in it imaginatively. It means getting rid of that vulnerability, yanking the patient out of it when you can. That was my job, wasn't it, especially in matters of life and death? Kindness is a form of respect, but medical care requires action. I couldn't share Beatriz's vulnerability any longer.

I needed her to be perfect with her pills, but I was imperfect with my words.

Although I was full of care, I was careless. I indulged myself, I faltered, I tried to humiliate her, and I was memorably unkind. Kindness is prone to collapsing, falling apart. It should be easy in the practice of medicine; the foundation of kindness is dependence, and the patient needs you. I understood Beatriz's consistent nonadherence as a sign that she didn't need me. Compassion is easiest with those who return the favor.

Her understanding of our silent contract, set early in our relationship, included three clauses: Don't mention HIV in front of my daughter; I'm going to be nonadherent with my medication; I will continue to come see you. I tried to change the contract. Hoping for a different, longer life for Beatriz, maybe I was the one with the magical thinking. In the end, it was her choice.

3

Acting like a Doctor

Dr. Helena Veri, a consultant, traveled the country helping doctors with what she called Being Clear. She was in her early forties, and her hair, parted in the center, reached her shoulders with an enthusiastic flip.

"You, in this room, have a communication problem," Dr. Veri said to our group of thirty primary care doctors gathered in a basement conference space for our usual 7 A.M. meeting that month. Our hospital, she told us, was among the lowest 10 percent of hospitals nationwide in patient-doctor satisfaction scores; this finding was the reason she had come to town. In the past, early morning group meetings had generally dealt with hospital reorganization concerns, new documentation requirements, practice plan mergers, insurance company reimbursement declines, the annual update regarding the overall budget and financial health of the organization—in sum, the latest changes in an increasingly chaotic world of health care. "Communication Quality," the subject of my email invitation this month, was a new and unusual topic.

She moved to her computer, set on a table in the middle of the room, and projected the first video clip onto a screen at the front. From the lower edge of the screen, a doctor approached a middle-aged man lying flat on his back on a stretcher and the woman in the low chair beside him. The video, while grainy, looked real (not actors simulating an encounter) with its half-pulled ceiling-to-floor curtain and the standard emergency department equipment (blood pressure cuff, ophthalmoscope, oxygen flow tube) on the wall behind the patient's head. Once settled at the foot of the stretcher, the doctor didn't address the woman or even acknowledge her, let alone ask who she was (wife? sister?), nor sit the patient up so they might see eye to eye on the same level. Instead, he quickly explained the tests he'd ordered, spoke fast, used jargon, and left no time for questions before dashing off. Veri showed three other videos, each with a "communication problem," that included scenes with old and young doctors, female and male patients, emergency room or outpatient settings; all of the visits were brief and rushed, some interrupted by nursing staff walking into the screen, some cut short by beepers going off.

I'm sure I was not alone in thinking, *She's stacked the deck; she's showing us the worst cases of lousy doctoring; I'm not like that.*

During the conversation that followed, we ridiculed the obviously incompetent physicians and wondered about patients' diagnoses. Yet our group's general conclusion after watching Veri's videotapes was *There's not enough time to get all our work done and be universally nice.* We were thinking about the day's upcoming patients.

She was ready for this objection. Don't just show us the problems, Veri knew we would insist: give us the answers you've been brought to town to provide, as concretely as possible. "I'm here to offer you a set of tools and strategies for structured communication, for Being Clear," she said. "These scripts will begin to solve your satisfaction problem. You should know that the leaders of your practice have decided that in the near future, your patients' satisfaction survey responses will be used to incentivize you financially."

I should have known that even a Communication Quality meeting would eventually lead back to money. I turned and looked longingly at the muffins on the table against the back wall.

She handed us a short stack of laminated index cards. "These are essential elements of communication. They are also basic manners," she said. It was difficult for us not to get our backs up when we were spoken to like children. It was mind-boggling that we needed this redress after years of seeing patients. She said, "See which ones resonate with you. Try some out with your patients. Come back in a week and let me know if they were helpful." Did she know we were annoyed? Is that why she ended our first session with her then, leaving us to go through these cards on our own?

The medical school where I teach instructs students how to behave in clinical settings by first sending them to see patients who aren't really patients but instead are paid medical actors, professionals hired to perform illness in staged classrooms. Wearing cotton gowns and presenting fictional lives and symptoms, these "standardized patients" know where it hurts and how to express it according to scripts they've been given—the single woman lawyer with seizures and a tranquilizer problem, the building manager with painless stomach ulcers and shortness of breath from anemia. (I'd thought of these scenarios when Veri ran through her videos.)

Playing along that these are real patients, the student goes on a diagnostic treasure hunt following a standard information-gathering protocol, an elaborate checklist of problems, practiced at home with classmates and friends. Organized to collect a reproducible narrative—why are you here, tell me the history of this complaint and your medical history more generally—the student is taught to move through the memorized catalog of symptoms—fatigue, fever, weakness, trouble sleeping, skin rash, hair or nail changes, and so on—a list of what can go wrong with a body. The student has fifteen minutes per patient, which enforces a galloping pace through the questions and a need to disguise the time pressure as true interest.

The student checklist prescribes certain actions—"Put the patient at ease," "Ensure patient readiness and comfort," "Comment on some personal quality or observation about the patient to elicit rapport"—that might already come naturally if they weren't on a checklist. These standardized actions have must been added since my training (we had also memorized only question lists when I was in school), because the latest generation of students wasn't doing so well during clinical visits. In these simulation exercises with pseudo patients, the student must try to remember these fundamental skills of social interaction—ask the patient for a name, sit down, make eye contact—in the nervousness of a first medical encounter, at the same time as she or he hones diagnostic skills. They are reminders to be human.

What's meant to be taught to the student through such encounters with mock patients is not only the branching symptom questions that lead to diagnosis, but also kindness. In the best case, students must be mindful that their questions are intrusive while they create an atmosphere that allows the vulnerable patient to tell the truth to a stranger. At the end of the interaction, the mock patient offers feedback to the student about how it felt to be examined, about the questions asked and the manner of asking, about helpful words and words that were awkward or constraining or rude. The exchange is videotaped through a one-way mirror so that the student can later watch his or her performance. The actor-patient completes a scorecard and writes a report—a satisfaction survey, as it were.

Of course, sitting with any patient is a complicated piece of theater: the lights, the costumes, giving them what you think they need, protecting yourself, controlling the outcome. A great stage or screen actor is not putting something *on* so much as *being*. To be convincing, the actor must link emotional moments from his life with that of his character so as to become that character. A doctor too is expected to carry an expanded emotional spectrum from his life as a doctor who has seen thousands of patients;

indeed, this is the source of his imaginative sympathy. He must have the emotional control and manipulation techniques familiar to an actor (who works from a script).

The doctor's patient is his costar, but also his audience. She is acting too; she is considering how to present herself, how to be taken seriously. She also exercises the demands of an audience, sitting before the doctor with her wounds, memories, agony; she wants her visit to be a self-revelation and an education in herself. She hopes her doctor notices and knows her, but also that he knows what's going on in her body and shares the news, even if he wears a mask and a white coat.

From the beginning of my medical training decades earlier, I understood, there was acting. On my first day with real patients as third-year medical student at Harlem Hospital, I had to pretend that I was competent. Everything was new then, every patient produced a fresh response in me and my peers, but we presented ourselves as more knowledgeable than we were. We had to pretend we knew how to talk on rounds, with patients, to nurses and families. My classmates and I had been coached, as a group, on how to present a case quickly (history, exam, lab testing, plan) in order to be of use to the senior doctors, the ones in the long white coats; our coats were shorter, the sign that we hadn't been doing this for as many years as they had. We did what our superiors told us to do; we acted respectful, even to the bastards. But we couldn't wait to be on our own.

Within a week, we'd learned that what patients told us was often wrong, or quite different from what they would tell the next person who interviewed them. We'd take a history, and then our professor would take the same history and gather completely different facts, as if we hadn't been listening or couldn't reliably repeat the simple answers we'd heard. This reversal was a common embarrassment for us. We were surprised the first and second time it happened, but we only acted surprised by the third time. This was apprenticeship, and we were like actors researching our parts.

We were tired, and we didn't have time to eat or play or see friends after work. We acted as if we were not angry that we were indentured. We acted as if we could still function at a high level at home in the evening, when during the day we tied patients into restraints, and hurt some. We acted as if none of this bothered us. We learned to do what we had to do. Admit to a semiprivate room, send for procedures, review results and diagnose, medicate, do surgery, plan for discharge. We started out idealistic, and then we began to cut our losses and only acted idealistic when we were talking to professors who rated us, or to our parents. We got used to being understudies who looked forward to performing well when the time came and we'd be given the lead. We hoped to know enough, to be confident enough, that our patients wouldn't know we were acting. But we began to question: If they knew, would they have cared?

When I am with patients, I sometimes still feel as if I'm acting, that every consultation is a kind of theater. The patient has the "sick" role, what sociologist Talcott Parsons described as a temporary, medically sanctioned form of deviant behavior.

Acting like a Doctor

Opposite them, I have to appear healthy (patients distrust doctors who are overweight or who smoke), caring, and involved, no matter how I feel, even if my son was suspended from school that morning, the cat escaped yesterday, my nephew's Marine unit was in a firefight last night, or my throat is sore. To be a doctor, to put on the long white coat, is to take on a role, to become a version of myself—or many versions over the course of a clinical day. With one patient I must have a skeptical fury at a specialist's advice; with the next I try hard to be relentlessly positive despite an ominous biopsy result. I never feel that I disappear into each version or character like a Method actor, as much as perform as any professional would if hired for a single, recurring performance. But I sometimes wonder: If the goal is to make the patient feel they've been given the attention they need, then is the best doctoring, the best communicating, a matter of force of personality, interest, and charisma, or can it be reflexive, practiced, and mechanical?

When Veri finished with her videos that first session, I'd bristled because I thought we were all far enough beyond our training, and teaching in an enlightened school, that we didn't need her services.

The scripts Veri handed us, one to a card, were key phrases to use at key times. The scripts informed us about how we were to speak to patients. "You can do it better than you have been," Veri said, as she passed around the rubber-banded stack of cards.

Which is another way of saying we weren't doing it right. The scripts were clearly directed at the friendliness and courtesy questions from our patient satisfaction survey.

On an initial greeting:

"I'm sorry for any wait you had. How can I best help you?"

"Sorry that you're in so much pain. Let's see how we can get you feeling better."

While listening to express concern:

"This must have been very difficult for you."

"You've been through a lot."

During the exam, offering reassurances:

"Your lungs sound clear."

"Your heart rhythm is steady."

When outlining what you propose:

"Let me describe what I have in mind, based on what you've told me, and you can tell me how it sounds to you."

"I'm going to suggest some options for what I think the next steps could be, and why, and you should let me know if it makes sense to you."

In closing:

"Have I forgotten anything?"

"Is there anything else you were hoping I could do for you today?"

Are scripts, delivered with feeling, the technique we must master to cope with the psychological demands of a rushed profession? Is learning to speak a script convincingly a skill equivalent to learning to read an X-ray, one gathering information from a person, the other from a machine?

I didn't think of myself as having a communication quality problem, but I became self-conscious when I sat in front of my first patient the day following our initial meeting with Veri. I wanted to be open-minded about Veri's cue cards for kindness, but I was unsettled by them. They made me think of something I'd overheard a colleague say to a group of medical students a few days earlier: "During training you become a professional doctor and an amateur human being."

When I started to say to my patient, "That must have been very difficult for you," I hesitated. I worried that the patient, who had been telling me about her faints, sudden hospitalization, and pacemaker insertion, whom I'd known for many years, would see through me because these were not words I'd ever used. I wondered what exactly the problem was that Veri's script was trying to fix: that doctors were likely to say too much or too little in an attempt to cover the awkwardness and enormity of the moments when illness is inflicting misery on patients?

Perhaps the goal of Veri's script was less about kindness than it was about avoiding saying something unkind. Because we would be working from a script, the words were supposedly focus-group-tested, mistake-proof. I got it. Patients had long memories of bad medical conversations, memories of ungenerous interactions. I thought of my sister's report of her recent visit to a dermatologist. She had gone to discuss a new treatment for her midlife psoriasis that had been triggered by a strep throat that did not respond as promised to standard therapies. She called me as soon as she got home. "Eight-minute appointment. He never addressed me by my name. He never looked me in the eye. He kept his eyes on my skin. He never said, 'How are you doing with all this? How's your mood been?' I was simply a body. I could have been *any* body. Not a person, a body, waiting to be told what to do. Not even a body, a collection of red spots. So he told me what drug to take next, without giving me the time to ask a question or make a decision about whether to accept. I guess all skin doctors are superficial," she said sarcastically.

If my sister had been sent a satisfaction survey she could have had her revenge by giving this doctor low ratings. For the medical student, learning a script was a defense against self-doubt, but also a kind of license: you know you will always have something to say in the emotion-filled moments that will inevitably arrive in your office. But for my sister's dermatologist, and perhaps for me, I understood that a scripted, stock, positively worded phrase was also perhaps a form of malpractice insurance.

Veri referred to "basic manners" in her presentation, but she did not use the word "kind." She did not use it to inspire our room full of doctors, as in, "Try to be kind when you have to deliver bad news." In fact, "kindness" was not included in any of the thirty satisfaction survey items our hospital collected, nor were any of the other names kindness goes by—"sympathy," "generosity," "benevolence," "compassion," "empathy." The questions in the survey that had placed our institution in the bottom 10 percent of hospitals nationwide (one produced and analyzed by a large consumer satisfaction conglomerate that had questions about the doctor's attitude toward patient requests, about skill) worked their way around the idea of kindness—"concern for your questions and worries," "friendliness/courtesy"—but didn't quite get there. "Did the staff work together to care for you?" Here the word "care" sounded utilitarian, Walmart-ian, not compassionate or empathetic—or kind. "To care for you" implied providing a patient with a competent, timely, efficient encounter and a smooth release back into the world. Was it too old-fashioned a word, a leftover from the days of house calls? Was it too abstract, too difficult to measure? Or, finally, was kindness not mentioned in our satisfaction survey because it was irrelevant?

Perhaps, said convincingly, "This must have been very difficult for you" may be understood as a kindness.

There are certainly situations where the doctor's very act of providing *complete* information during a visit increases the patient's perception of the physician as compassionate, caring, and empathetic, and there is research to show that it is this *perception* of completeness, not the facts provided, that relieves a patient's anxiety. Is satisfaction the reduction of anxiety during the medical visit? Is that what's remembered and transformed into the responses on satisfaction surveys?

I had a friend who at the time of her newly diagnosed pancreatic cancer asked her doctor what she could hope for. "A miracle," he said. She pressed him: "Prognostically, how long do I have?" She knew it wasn't long, months, maybe a few years. He couldn't, or wouldn't, tell her. Everyone's different, he said, but some treatment, palliative, not curative, would make it longer. Was this an example of providing complete information? Yes, if we expect doctors to know the future. Was it a satisfactory answer? For her, that day, it was.

Veri's suggestion that even short, rote statements—forty seconds' worth, or maybe even less—affect the patient's experience has empirical support. An experiment was designed almost two decades ago to vary perceptions of a physician's compassion by varying the methods that express support, sympathy, and compassion for a patient's difficult situation both in words and by touch. Oncologists were videotaped offering consultations to advanced breast cancer patients regarding a new treatment. Five common components from these conversations were extracted: an introduction, a summary of previous treatment, the objective of the new treatment, a discussion of treatment risks and benefits, and treatment alternatives. The researchers then wrote a script that included the best of all five components, using a pastiche of the oncologists' own words. They then recorded a master videotape with another oncologist acting the part of the physician and reciting the prepared script to a woman, who had not had cancer previously, acting the part of the patient. The dramatized tape of an oncologist talking to a breast cancer patient tape lasted approximately eighteen minutes. The researchers edited two versions of this dramatized scene to be tested against one another, measuring a viewer's sense of the physician.

In the "standard" videotape version, the physician described two options for metastatic breast cancer, high-dose chemotherapy and low-dose chemotherapy, using the five components. The "enhanced compassion" videotape was identical to the standard videotape (i.e., the same footage was used) except for the addition of two short segments. In these two segments, the oncologist acknowledged the psychological concerns of the patient, expressed partnership and support, validated her emotional state and the difficulty of making a decision, touched her hand, and tried to reassure her. The brief segments were:

(1) I know this is a tough experience to go through, and I want you to know that I am here with you. Some of the things that I say to you today may be difficult to understand, so I want you to feel comfortable in stopping me if something I say is confusing or doesn't make sense. We are here together, and we will go through this together.

(2) I know this is a tough time for you, and I want to emphasize again that we are in this together. I will be with you each step along the way.

Segment 1 appeared near the beginning of the videotape, before the physician provided treatment information. Segment 2 came close to the end of the consultation. The two segments added exactly forty seconds to the videotape.

Both breast cancer survivors and women who had never had cancer were recruited to view the videotapes and answer questions about the doctor-patient interaction. Participants rated the physician's compassion using five pairs of physician characteristics, each rated from 0 to 100. The characteristics were "warm/

cold," "pleasant/unpleasant," "compassionate/distant," "sensitive/insensitive," and "caring/uncaring."

When the physician acknowledged the patient's emotional state during the forty seconds of "enhanced" compassion (segment 2) in the course of an eighteen-minute visit, viewers perceived this physician as significantly more empathetic than the "standard." In addition, the more compassionate physician was also rated higher on wanting what was best for the patient, caring about the patient, acknowledging the patient's emotions, encouraging questions, and encouraging involvement in decision-making. As one viewer put it: "It's not that he'll treat you better. It's like a backstage pass. The show's the same. You're just closer."

Just like it is the *perception* of completeness that matters, it is the *perception* of compassion that matters. Studies indicate that this sense that your physician is compassionate is directly related to patient satisfaction.

As a good consultant, Veri had constructed a way to manipulate patient perception. To produce consistent and excellent results day after day, to reduce the avoidable error of turning patients off inadvertently during office visits, her Being Clear scripts might help. The scripts would not be foolproof at catching communication lapses (grimacing, sarcasm, slips of the tongue, patient misinterpretations), but they were a defense against fatigue and inattention and forgetfulness. They were bolsters for the bottom 10 percent.

An office visit is a delicate emotional play that comes to neither a tragic nor a happy ending. If the doctor does her job during their time together, the patient feels he's told a story that makes him visible to himself, a portrait his doctor has seen clearly, and he understands the options available to make him better, or make him feel better. The doctor has shared some news the patient didn't know on the way into the office.

Would Veri's formula, with these simple statements of solidarity, fulfill what patients expect? Could her plan, which ensured forty seconds of compassion, ensure that patients will not feel disappointed? Her scripts offered no promise of a cure, just a good-faith process to keep the patient feeling the doctor cares. Would this be enough? Or is satisfaction more closely related to outcome (splint applied painlessly, heart attack prevented, psoriasis gone) as the student in his simulation exercise believed?

The playacting of the doctor is the opposite of Method acting—his words are often *not* an extension of his emotional state. Reciting a script, no matter how artfully performed, does not depend on how the doctor feels; a script provides the illusion of feeling. This acting, the emotional labor of doctoring, brief for surgeons who focus on manual labor, is extended for psychiatrists who must engage a vital part of themselves with every interaction, but who know better than most that perhaps it's sometimes best not to say anything.

Acting like a doctor requires a repertoire of performances desired or demanded in a particular situation at a particular time. Is being able to act well a selling out, a betrayal of my "authentic self," or a sign of virtuosity? What's wrong with wanting to please? After all, patients are comparing my performance with the performance of other doctors and with the wished-for doctor in their minds.

Yet I refused to believe that mechanical empathy, written out on slick laminated cards, could produce the perception of caring. There had to be room to individualize (an actor would say ad lib) with the patient in front of you. Actually caring, instead of just impersonating a caring doctor, was what mattered. Said repeatedly, scripts might begin to move the amateur human being into a full and alert human being, but I didn't want to think of myself as an amateur.

At the start of our second session, Veri projected the phrases we were to have used during the past week as we flipped through the cards she'd provided at the first session. She wanted to know which ones were helpful, how the week had gone, what had changed. I was thinking: Should we admit, as doctors, that we're playacting? Does this acting create an unsupportable tension with the scientific truth we are there to transmit? Do patients want us to act? Do they care? Could they even tell? Maybe scripts *are* the right approach for amateur human beings, and if you believe that medical training turns too many who enter the field into amateurs, then scripts may indeed improve those in the bottom 10 percent. Yet I suspect that if I were to say the same thing many times, even the illusion of feeling would get refined out of it.

I was silent during this second meeting with Veri. At the end I dramatically tossed her index cards in the garbage on the way out.

Why was I so angry? Because I believed that day, and still believe, that there are visits where the doctor is polite, makes good eye contact, does not rush, is courteous, yet remains somehow neglectful. Because, as a romantic, I believe in kindness, which starts with, but is different from, civility. Kindness occurs when some existential dimension of a patient's suffering that *needs* to be touched *is* touched. Because I don't want to be told what to say to be human. Because I don't want to feel, after all these years, like I still have to act as I did when I was a student at Harlem Hospital.

I was upset, but I was also dismayed. It was sad to me that any group of doctors needed index cards to be kind.

Kindness and unkindness occur, notably, in times of uncertainty, and most medical visits are loaded with uncertainty, on both sides, about what we will hear or say. Kindness occurs when a doctor lets his patient know, "You're in the middle of something of impact; nothing you say is foolish." The risk of a script is that it becomes a coerced, mechanical response. The risk of a script is that it becomes tired, redundant, and the patient feels that he is one among many, not the one who needs treatment now.

Kindness appears at the intersection of randomness and alertness, those unplanned moments when I am unprepared for what I hear and feel from a patient. Perceived as a duty, the precise, explicit conversational plan of a script precludes these unplanned moments, and without the possibility of surprise, there is little reason to listen carefully. The risk of a script is that the doctor stops listening because his responses are already programmed, because his next words could be applied to any patient, because he's said them all before.

When am I dissatisfied as a patient? My answer is the same as my sister's: when I am not listened to; when the responses I receive from my doctor are rote, thoughtless, and impersonal though we are talking about the most personal things in my life.

There is drama to being a doctor. At its best, doctoring is a specific form of impersonation, or in-personation. It is when I take a patient's passion (her pain, her complaint) within myself for a few seconds. When the disorder of a meandering conversation pulls me into the patient's story, making *their* story *my* story, and seeing it through their eyes begins to create order in me. It is a kind of self-transformation. It can't be acted. It lies in some deeper script indelibly written in the nervous system, connecting astonishment and gratification.

4

Full Hearted and Half Empty

I sometimes referred my patients to a cardiologist who was a classmate of mine in medical school, Paul Dinnell, who happened to have landed in the same hospital where I worked. Although we'd never become friends socially during the twenty years we'd lived in neighboring towns, I'd always admired his work habits, the clear thought processes he described in his chart notes, the outcomes of his procedures. He was good with his hands; he built twenty-four-foot wooden sailboats in his garage with his sons and piloted them along our famous coastline. Patients I referred to him liked him.

Whenever I saw Paul, I was reminded of something he'd said to me during the first year of medical school when we were taking Anatomy. His father was a family doctor in a small rural town in West Virginia. "I've seen this kind of destruction before," Paul said as we stood outside the anatomy lab where, over the course of that year, we would hemisect and work on the decapitated head of a cadaver. "One thing I learned growing up, hanging around my father's office, was that if I could hang on when I saw the blood, I liked the feeling of being able to dissociate myself enough to be able to function. My father noticed too. When he dropped me off at college, he said that being the unflappable one in a crowd ought to be put to some good, and maybe I should consider medicine."

As opposed to "sympathy" (which means "pity" or "compassion"), "empathy," since the nineteenth century, has been a larger concept referring to the mutual sharing of feelings among people—"fellow feeling." Doctors who do "people work" of some kind like to think we have a special sense of empathy, an instinctive identification with the vulnerability of others. We wouldn't like to think of ourselves as professional mourners, people hired to cry at funerals. Rather, our emotional life evolves under the direct influence of the feelings of those around us, those we care for. We are "taken out of ourselves" into the emotional world of others, as Hume wrote. When we see pain, we feel pain.

This is not only true of doctors. But we like to think of doctors (and nurses) as particularly openhearted and compassionate. The empathetic medical self is an expansive self, one for whom the happiness of others is the sine qua non of our own well-being. If you are incapable of empathetic identification, you are inhuman—a Dr. Frankenstein in the nineteenth century, a computer today.

However, I sometimes wonder whether the people drawn to medicine—those who have the quality of unflappability described by Paul's father—are in some sense naturally less empathetic. Or whether being a good doctor requires, at the least, training yourself to exhibit less empathy than normal. But if so, what are the costs of doing this, and how can we measure them? And what happens when a doctor gets exhausted from the effort of trying to feel less?

One of the patients I referred to Paul was a man named Kadden. I'd met Kadden first in my office fifteen years before when he came in with a painful left hip. Twelve years later I'd diagnosed him with chronic leukemia, and he'd been on one or another form of chemotherapy ever since. Now he was in the hospital again, a week after Thanksgiving, arriving the day of the winter's first snowfall.

It wasn't really a question—was it?—if I knew the answer before asking, but as I stood at the foot of his bed, I asked anyway: "How are you?"

"I seem to have leukemia today." He'd had it every day for three years, and he smilingly offered this health report as if it was news every time I saw him.

He was charming and funny, seventy-one and dying. His lips were colorless, with white specks at the corner. I hadn't seen him in a while, about six months. As his primary care doctor, I'd mostly handed him over to the oncologists after the leukemia infiltrated the lymph nodes of his neck. They had created serial cocktails of chemo that weren't working too well anymore.

He'd come in to the hospital that morning with a vague jaw discomfort. The cancer specialists had decided that his symptom had nothing to do with leukemia and that therefore *I* should take over his care during his stay as we worked toward a diagnosis.

I didn't remember Kadden's body when I examined it in his hospital bed. He'd lost eighteen pounds in the last six months and was far thinner than he'd been a decade and a half earlier.

"You told me yourself, you never learn much from the exam. It's all in the history, you said. So why are you bothering?" he asked, teasing me.

My hands crawled over him, poking. His ribs were ladders. His shoulders felt like a steering wheel in my grip. His muscles had receded. I could see individual gray hairs in his eyebrows. The lymph nodes in his groin were pebbly again, abnormal. I thought about how little I knew him or his body anymore. I did not know him as a body that stepped into baths, danced at weddings, ate in restaurants, squeezed into tuxedoes, stood in a shower, stretched, jumped, dug for worms, got in line at the market, typed, threw Frisbees and baseballs, sat through bad movies, turned a wrench, pulled in a fishing line, pushed a chess piece, crammed into a bus seat in another country. I knew him only in the confines of my office exam room and knew his body as a series of thickenings and thinnings, nodules, discolorations, and other troubles.

Before this episode of jaw pain and sudden sweating, I'd heard he wasn't doing well. He was between courses of chemotherapy, and the next regimen would be extremely toxic. With his new fatigue and weight loss, he was considering whether he wanted to bother with another round of chemo. It was more likely that if he needed hospitalization, it would be for a leukemia-related complication, under the care of his oncology team, yet here he was with a nonleukemic problem.

I suspected that the ache in his jaw more likely came from blocked coronary arteries in this man who'd smoked Marlboros for thirty years while he was a newspaper editor. He hadn't suffered a heart attack, but his jaw pain and the sweating were harbingers.

Paul was convinced that the pain, along with Kadden's risk factors and his abnormal EKG, made the likelihood of severe blockage high, and he arranged for a heart catheterization the following afternoon. He wanted to see the anatomy so he could lay out the treatment options and describe the urgency.

Afterward, back in Kadden's room, I was there when Paul made a pencil drawing of the heart on the back of the hospital menu, diagramming the four blocked arteries, including the largest, the main feeder, a lousy finding.

"Why do they keep these rooms so dark?" Kadden asked, reaching for his glasses, which I pushed across the plastic levitating breakfast table to him. "It's like permanent evening here."

Kadden was one of those patients all doctors like. With an easy laugh, he was obviously ready for whatever it was you wanted to do with him. Now he knew how bad his heart condition was despite changing the subject to the room lighting. I felt bad for him.

***

Here are the items from the Personal Accomplishment Inventory, published in the *Journal of Occupational Behavior*, part of a scale developed by researchers to help those in the "human service institutions" assess their feelings about themselves on the job:

I can easily create a relaxed atmosphere with my clients.
I feel exhilarated after working closely with my clients.
I have accomplished many worthwhile things in this job.
In my work, I deal with emotional problems very calmly.

Each statement is rated on two dimensions: frequency and intensity. Frequency ranges from "Never" to "Every day." When administered to a range of professionals—police, teachers, lawyers (substituting "clients" or "students" for "patients")—very few individuals responded "Never" to any of these.

Although I have a tendency to evaluate myself negatively, particularly in regard to my work, in the hours after I first saw Kadden in the hospital, I would have said "every day" to each of these statements. My high score on the Personal Accomplishment Inventory that December I would have provided an evaluator with unambiguous evidence of my high morale. I would have openly and strongly resisted any suggestion of job dissatisfaction, even though I'd had a difficult few months—one of my patients had overdosed, another lost a child to angiosarcoma, a third died of liver failure—and even though that Friday I remember being annoyed that Kadden's arrival would complicate a weekend I expected to be quiet.

Here are some of the items from the Emotional Exhaustion Inventory:

I feel emotionally drained from my work.

I feel used up at the end of the workday.

I feel fatigued when I get up in the morning
    and have to face another day on the job.

I feel frustrated by my job.

I feel I'm working too hard on my job.

I feel I'm at the end of my rope.

I would have disagreed with every one of them on the day Kadden came in. Or perhaps I would have answered, "Who doesn't from time to time?"

I felt a special kinship with Kadden. I found his self-deprecating humor vital, liberating, a call to life. I was inappropriately hopeful for him, given his medical problems. I wanted him to do inordinately well.

A recent experiment: while lying in an fMRI scanner to measure the activation of specific regions of your brain, you are shown video clips of the faces of persons who are described as patients suffering from a neurological disease affecting their hearing, a kind of tinnitus. The videos are shot against a light blue curtain you'd see in a hospital, with actor-patients wearing white gowns and large headphones. At certain times, the patients lower their brows, squeeze their eyes shut, mouth curses, and press their lips tightly, all signals of distress. You're told that these patients are undergoing a new therapy consisting of repeated sounds of specific frequencies and amplitudes that result in great pain but may improve hearing in the long run. You get to hear a sample of these awful sounds but are made aware that the pain evoked in the video patients is considerably stronger due to their neurological illness.

When watching the video, you are asked to rate the degree of the witnessed pain and your own feelings of discomfort. Then you are shown a second video and asked to imagine how you would feel *if you were in the place of the wincing patient.* These two responses require distinct forms of perspective-taking that likely carry different emotional consequences, which may originate from different sites in the brain. The former usually evokes empathetic concern (an other-oriented response congruent with the perceived distress of the person in pain), whereas the latter induces personal distress (i.e., a self-oriented emotional response—"I want this to stop, I want to get away").

Both the self-perspective and the other-perspective turn out to be associated with activation in the neural network involved in pain processing—the same areas that activate when you are stuck with a needle—including the parietal operculum, the anterior insula, but also the anterior medial cingulate cortex, the part of the brain that prepares for a behavioral response, getting you ready to escape pain. When witnessing the pain of others, we may be aware of our own discomfort—there is affective sharing, an emotional contagion—or we may not; we may repress it so that this brain activity never reaches consciousness.

You are then told that the video clips of the neurological patients include two groups of individuals. You are told that because this new sound therapy is being used for the first time, some of the patients may benefit from it, while others will not.

The goal of this experiment is to assess the respective contribution of two processes that influence *how much* empathy one feels: the contribution of perspective-taking (self vs. other, as in the experiment with the first two videos), and additionally, the contribution of cognitive appraisal, that is the effect of taking into account the different treatment implication for the patient.

Adopting the perspective of the *other* evoked strong empathetic concern, whereas personal distress was higher when imagining oneself to be in the painful situation. Witnessing another person suffering and knowing that the treatment had not been effective increased emotional distress in the observer, and knowing the treatment had been effective decreased the viewer's distress. This might indicate that participants focused not solely on the sensory aspects of the observed pain but also on its ultimate unpleasantness or "badness," taking into account the long-term consequences for the patient.

The observation of pain in others and of experiencing it oneself activate a largely overlapping neural-emotional network. When I say, "I feel your pain," I am describing, literally, what is happening in the pain pathways of *my* brain. But there are other brain areas silently turned on as one watches the video clips of the faces of the patients suffering a neurological disease affecting their hearing. The brain areas that generate movement are also activated. Why? What parts of the body get prepared to move when witnessing pain?

There are two. The brain region that controls the muscles of your face activate such that you can mirror the facial pain expressions displayed by the person in the video. Your facial movements can be subtle, invisible to the eye. But this motor mimicry is more overt and pronounced when you're asked, "How would you yourself feel if you were in the place of the patient?" The second brain region that is prompted has to do with the movement required if you were about to withdraw from pain—the hand and leg regions are activated. This mimicking, what brain scientists call "inverse mapping," is automatic and unconscious.

Perhaps this is what we mean when we say we were "moved" by another's pain; more accurately, we are ready to move. Our empathetic response is brain-embedded and mixed in with our mechanisms of self-protection.

Paul added a few more medications to Kadden's daily diet and recommended bypass surgery; the medication-only option was suboptimal, he reported, and the blockages were unreachable with stents. The morning following the procedure, on Sunday, December 3, when I was eating cornbread and honey at home, Kadden had another episode of jaw pain, along with pain in his left scapula and some nausea. The hospital team added yet another heart medication to his list.

"At home, when you're feeling pretty good and going through your day, you have to remember to worry. Here, you have to tell yourself not to worry," Kadden said to me on Monday morning.

He'd ordered double dessert the evening before, he informed me: chocolate pudding and lemon meringue pie. He shared them with his wife. "Sunday night is date night," he said ironically.

Paul had recommended a big surgery. The thoracic specialists had gotten better at open-heart procedures over the past few decades, but there was still the risk of stroke and paralysis and never waking up at all after the bypass, he told Kadden.

Kadden asked me what I thought about his having the operation. Patients looked to me for guidance. I was supposed to give advice, even when there was really no good advice to give. But in Kadden's case, the path was obvious. Heart disease was fixable, and doctors know how to fix it; Kadden's problem was knowable and correctable; surgery could bypass the unstentable difficulties. "Have the surgery," I said.

I kept thinking of my father. Kadden's illness brought back memories of my father's final days, and by association, I didn't want to let Kadden die as I'd "let" my father die of heart disease when I was thirteen. I had the opportunity to keep Kadden from dying (at least for a while) if I did my job now that he'd come into the hospital. I noticed as I'd left Kadden's room that despite his bravado, he'd looked twice at his IV, the way a man double-checks the lock on his door.

All empathy is self-pity, D. H. Lawrence remarked, formulating a particular suspicion of kindness: kindness as a higher form of selfishness, one that is morally triumphant and secretly exploitative.

On Monday evening, when I came around again, I offered Kadden, who was uncertain, an exaggerated and frightening summary I'd heard one or another cardiologist (not Paul) say to patients who needed a push toward a heart procedure:

"You have a time bomb in your chest."
"Your luck could run out."
"Think of your wife: the narrowing of
    that vessel is a widow maker."
"I'm frightened by your anatomy."
"You could die at any moment."
"You're in big trouble."
"You could have a heart attack at any time."
"The surgery should have been done yesterday."

Each applied to Kadden, and I said all of them. It was a brutal assault.

Here are the items of the Depersonalization Inventory from the same scale:

I feel I treat some patients as if they were impersonal objects.
I've become more callous toward people since I took this job.
I worry this job is hardening me emotionally.
I don't really care what happens to some patients.

How would any doctor answer these questions? How would I have answered that day? I would have disagreed with every one, or if given a chance to include a freehand response to each, I would have written: "Never."

Any increase in callousness occurred during medical train-ing, long before this job. I didn't think of myself as hardened, but I was often worried about it.

Frankness is not kindness. Driving a patient to despair by making him imagine the worst is unkind.

I shivered. What I said to him last was untrue. "You have no choice but to have the operation." He did have a choice, but I had convinced myself that he didn't; I needed him to make the right decision.

The sense of omniscience is not part of the Depersonaliza-tion Inventory, but it should be.

A complete blurring of self and other is not the purpose of empa-thy. As Paul's father knew, we must have a way of not being overwhelmed as we go through the world experiencing the pain of others. Among various emotion regulation strategies when observing a person in pain, we must also be able to *deny* its direct relevance to us. This denial of relevance is what we mean when we say we are "detached." Detachment is the ability to generate an image of ourselves observing, and by doing so convince ourselves that we are unaffected by the person in pain. Such a strategy is likely to play an important role in preventing empathetic over-arousal and remaining within the finite economy of empathy.

When it became clear to researchers that perceiving the pain of others activates a large part of the pain centers in the observer, it became interesting to study the regulatory mechanism that must operate in people who see pain on a regular basis, or even more clearly, among doctors who *inflict* painful in their practice.

A study compared fourteen doctors who practice acupuncture with fourteen age-matched nondoctors who'd never seen or experienced acupuncture. Lying within MRI machines, brains being scanned, both groups watched video of either acupuncture needles pricking the hands, feet, and lips of patients or of Q-tips touching the same spots. During each set of videos (painful/nonpainful), the doctors and nondoctors were scanned.

Confirming the earlier study of painful sounds, there were again striking similarities in the neural circuits involved in the processing of both the firsthand experience of pain and by the sight of other persons in pain. The mere visualization of the expected pain from acupuncture needles led to a response in the brain's pain regions in the nondoctor viewers, a response not activated by watching the Q-tips videos. This is the brain scan version of empathy. In addition, these pain sensitivity regions (i.e., the anterior cingulate cortex and insula) were not equally activated in the doctor group. Instead, doctors rated painful situations as significantly less unpleasant and painful than the control participants did. The parahippocampal gyrus and right inferior parietal lobule were activated, regions of cognitive control and emotion regulation, regions that mediate the function of detachment.

If our sense of sharedness of feelings is absolute, if there is a complete overlap between ourselves and others, we would be distressed all the time; yet we must be able to toggle between a self-perspective and an other-perspective. Doctors who have expertise in acupuncture procedures know that such situations can be painful for their patients, but they have learned throughout their training and practice to inhibit the empathy pain response in the brain. These doctors have quieted the brain region that registers the pain of others while activating brain regions of cognitive control and emotion regulation, brain regions of detachment. It is sympathy without "fellow feeling." But how far is it from what we mean when we say someone has "shut down"?

Kadden was weak, his leukemia advancing. His chance of any response to chemotherapy was worsening. His enthusiasm had evaporated. But his mind was sharp. He'd scoured his thinking of everything extraneous. "Here's how I see it," Kadden said. "I have two options, neither one good. I can crawl either onto a ledge or into a cave. I can have surgery and chemo or I can go home for the countdown. I think I'll go home."

My job was to keep him alive. Or put another more truthful way, I didn't want him to die. Was it possible that I cared *too* much? Kadden's decision was unacceptable. He was sad about the situation, but he was also practical and had survival instincts; I thought I could change his mind.

That's when I moved beyond fearmongering and started my salesmanship, my seduction. The surgery wasn't so bad, I told Kadden; he'd feel lousy for four or five days, then only his chest wall would ache; then he would go home to his best slippers and cherry pie and grandchildren and his favorite sports on TV. With most patients my relationship was static, polite, superficial, pure, and simple, not a free-for-all where I attacked and forced the patient to parry. I didn't usually feel the need to reach down into my depths. I made a desperate effort with Kadden. I assumed this was the appropriate response to his condition. I did what I considered my job: I made a single-minded investment in his life.

I waited for his wife to come in. I'd missed every one of her visits before this one, and I was ready to pull her into his decision-making. In front of her, I again pitched him about the benefits of surgery, and he growled back at me.

"I know your approach. We're Americans—not passive. We must act when threatened, and I'm under threat."

"Exactly," I said.

"I thought doctors don't shout," he said. "Don't you take an oath about that?"

He didn't look at her. He was a bit afraid of her, as if she knew many embarrassing secrets about him. I imagined him at another time in his life smoking and arguing with someone at a party. In this scene she would be there waiting beside him, head down, listening silently until she was sick and tired of it, and then she would put her hand on his back, interrupting him in her low, decisive voice. "That's enough for tonight. Let's get going."

I wanted to say to her, Could you live with yourself if you woke up and your husband was lying dead at your side when you knew that surgery would have saved his life?

Her eyes stopped on my clipboard and then on my eyes. I thought, for a second, Now the three of us will have a real conversation about his heart where my omniscience and authority will win out, and he, with her urging, will do what I say to save himself. But there was no chance of that. In her eyes was a soft look. She turned back to her husband.

Kadden no longer had certain expectations. He seemed to know instinctively that patients often don't get as far as they had quite reasonably expected. It always seemed unfair. "The expression 'Whatever doesn't kill me makes me stronger' doesn't work in the hospital," he said. "There are plenty of things that could kill me here, and the ones that don't will certainly make me weaker."

"So why come to the hospital at all if you don't want our care?" I asked. It was a mean and unconscionable and unprofessional thing to say and did not absorb what he'd been through, his thoughtfulness about what lay ahead.

"If that's what you've decided, let's get you home," his wife said. Her face was pale and tense, but her tired green eyes, looking straight into his, held not a single tear.

The acupuncturists automatically activated the right temporal-parietal region, an area known to play an important role in self/other distinction. They'd trained their minds to remember that pain was happening to someone else when they placed their needles.

It seemed obvious that this unconscious self-regulation was necessary for successful professional practice. But what I thought when I first read this study was: Is this inhibition of the empathy pain response a specific response to work situations for these acupuncture doctors, or were these doctors generally, disposition-ally, less empathetic? Would acupuncture doctors have the same brain responses as nondoctors when witnessing other forms of pain they do not see everyday, for instance the pain of the sound therapy in the earlier experiment? Do doctors shut down their affective response because they learn that in some way or shape they are always causing or are about to cause or witness pain?

And then I wondered: Can the necessary inhibitory system get fatigued? Is there a point where we can no longer differentiate ourselves from others, and all our patients' pain is ours?

When I was in training, Dr. Albano was known for his aggres-sive approach. I was a resident helping him care for an emaciated man in his nineties who had metastatic cancer, and I was on call when the man developed a fever. On the phone, from home at 2 A.M., Albano told me to do a spinal tap to look for a treatable cause. Albano had good clinical skills and utter dedication; he always covered his own patients, every day of the year; medicine was his life. He had an ethical code for what doctors must do for patients. He tried to shame those who favored palliative care over prolongation of life at any cost. He had the intensity of someone with a calling. "Don't try to tell me what's best for my patient" was his refrain. His decisions had an air of urgency and necessity. When I told the old man with a fever what Albano suggested, the patient did not want to offend his doctor. He acceded to the test despite the pain it would cause.

Now I was Albano. My attempt to frighten Kadden by listing every bad outcome was a sign that I had shut off from his pain.

And in addition, I couldn't match my professor's power. I had failed to convince Kadden of anything.

"You're really a very good doctor in spite of all the people who say you're very good," Kadden said, trying to make me feel better before I left his room that final morning. He'd noticed I'd changed; I must have looked dismal and ruined.

But his compliment didn't make me feel better. Compassion is an unstable emotion. It needs to be translated into action or it deteriorates. If there's nothing you can do for a patient, you become mean, cynical.

Paul gave me a smile later that day when I told him about Kadden's decision. He wasn't upset like I was. His smile was not one of derision or contempt. It was not an ironic smile but a genuine one, a smile of wisdom and acceptance. A smile that said, "Of course, that's life, what else did you expect?"

I had *empathy* for Kadden, a kind of feeling with, a vicarious sharing of his feelings. He was sad, I was miserable. Had I lost the ability to quiet the brain region that registered the pain of others while activating brain regions of cognitive control and emotion regulation? Paul had *sympathy* for Kadden. He felt concern, he was motivated to alleviate Kadden's suffering, but he didn't feel sad or distressed by his patient's decision.

I was jealous of Paul as I had been outside the anatomy lab. I couldn't help myself. He'd always had and never lost the unconscious self-regulation that allows one to function.

On the face of it, true empathy is impossible, and to think otherwise is self-flattering. Kadden suffered alone. I didn't really *share* his feelings. I did not have to make his daily choice to go on, or not go on, with cancer, with heart disease.

For patients, much of illness involves the struggle to retain civility and kindness in the face of extraordinary pain and upset. I remember the day the leukemia report came back twelve years earlier, when Kadden first learned the bad news, heard the chemotherapy catalogue, and listened to the prognosis. After the shitstorm of news that was his new life, he said, "Anything else?" He refused to be cowed or fazed.

The day Kadden left the hospital to await death, I began to experience a mental winter. For weeks afterward I felt groggy. It was not a pensive mood that contained hope. It was a hollow mood, or shallow, without depth. I knew I was surely and direly ill suited for whatever the next weeks held and I had to make some changes in my work life. I tried to make myself feel something. Maybe not always a full-hearted response, but something.

I still went to my office and saw one patient and the one after that, and the one after that, but they felt unfamiliar and weirdly inaccessible. My examinations were rushed, cursory, anxious. I tried to appreciate some of the tragic joy of illness and recovery that patients brought to me during those weeks; I tried to empathize. But I had been uninvited from pleasure.

THE INVOLVEMENT INVENTORY

I feel similar to my patients in many ways.

I feel personally involved with my patients' problems.

Full Hearted and Half Empty

You are in trouble when your response moves from "Too much" to "Not at all." Burnout is not sadness—it is the refusal of sadness.

There was failure in the air. I had failed Kadden. I wanted to call him. I wanted to ask him how he was, but really I wanted to try to change his mind. I wanted to try to make him feel guilty for disappointing me.

How did I ever come to do this work, I asked myself. At one time it felt like an integral component of my life, but now it was unwelcome, superfluous, meaningless. My daily drive home, generally full of daydreams and reveries interspersed with remembered moments of particular patients from the day, and at times fresh insights and new ways of seeing, had only its opposite: a blankness. When I left the hospital those December evenings, I thought of nothing in particular, or I thought of Kadden. If I was lucky, I perseverated on another patient's pain—a woman who told me she'd had blood drawn so many times that each new needle felt like a pitchfork.

Kadden had decided there was nothing more I could do for him. Outside the car was a vast still space. Work was supposed to protect me from this strange, angry, featureless state.

You can't burn out unless you were once burning. And that is what empathy is, I've decided, a burning, a brain fire, a distress when the patient's pain is your pain, and both pains must constantly be quenched, which at certain times with certain patients, becomes impossible. Burnout is the extinction of empathy; it often begins as rage but is followed by the chill of detachment.

It is the cold perversion of caring, and it's only known afterward, not when it's happening. If I had had an fMRI, watching the videos of the neurology patients, every day during and in the days immediately after my time with Kadden, what would each have shown?

After Beatriz, after Kadden, I stopped working for a while, trying to understand what had happened to me. It took me time, months, to remember that this was work I'd always loved, that anyone would love. To understand that genuine connection was possible. The return of kindness—not deference, but a form of condolence, because kindness is a response to sadness—was the sign that I had again imaginatively identified with another's pain, which for a time would become my own, and I knew if I could keep from being burned, I would be redeemed.

5

Making Impressions

Not long ago, I was floundering around shaken by my mistakes with patients, wondering if I was a good doctor anymore, and feeling like I wasn't even sure what would constitute being a good doctor. I found myself thinking of the time when I had to choose doctors to care for me. What qualities did I look for?

I remembered the year that I turned forty-two and had to choose two doctors for myself. One was a neurosurgeon—I needed an operation for what I hoped would be a single, uncomplicated procedure to remove a tumor growing from my skull. The other was an internist—the kind of doctor I am—who would care for me when I went home after that surgery, and for years into the future. To answer a friend of mine, I've tried to understand how I picked my doctors. I wish I had used a brilliant and objective mechanism. I wish I had answered, "Choose the one you think is kindest." But it wasn't like that at all.

By my early forties I had been bald for a decade, so anyone looking could easily see the bump on the pale wide plain of my brow—any viewer, that is, except me. My wife had been the first to say something, brushing her finger over the pebble under my skin on the right side of my forehead just over the eyebrow. Then for the next twenty-four months I watched it grow into a smooth convexity, a thumb pushing out over the drum of my skull-skin. That is, I ignored it. I was like any patient: at the beginning of illness is the predominance of hope over knowledge.

I finally read up on the possible diagnoses of a bone-based tumor, of course, and only a few of them, the rarest on the list—the ones that were cancers, the ones that began in brain tissue and expanded with great force, the ones I'd convinced myself that I didn't have because I felt well—seemed serious enough to warrant getting evaluated, which I knew might mean a surgeon drilling into my head. Having ignored my lump for so long—it had become so familiar and prominent to my wife she called me "Lumpy"—I was slow to agree that I needed to have it investigated.

Because I had no doctor of my own, because I knew that the next step was a CT scan of my head, because I didn't want to wait once I'd decided to pay attention to my lump (and my wife), in an absolute breach of protocol, I asked one of my colleagues to order the scan for me. It showed the bone of my forehead holding a cherry-sized tumor pushing out through the thick resistant crust of my skull, while also expanding in toward the soft white folds of my now identifiably at-risk brain. I was angry at myself for delaying. I was embarrassed by my innocence. I was suddenly in a great hurry to know my diagnosis and treatment options.

Making Impressions

I made appointments with two neurosurgeons to decide which one—Dr. A or Dr. Z—should perform my operation. Both came highly recommended; I'd met Dr. A a few times over the years around my hospital; I'd never met Dr. Z. Dr. A's waiting room had light purple walls and oil paintings. In his converted factory building, there were tall windows without curtains, and spring afternoon light streamed onto wide carpets. Inside his office, Dr. A immediately offered bottles of water to me and my wife, and smiled. I didn't open my bottle, although my mouth was dry. My hands were too sweaty and I was trying, unsuccessfully, to concentrate on his mouth, which made words I was unable to follow, while my wife nodded. Unable to keep track of what he said, I tried to keep a list in my mind of what I noticed. His ears had black hairs inside, but his shave was extremely close. He wore a blue tie, and his cuff links tapped the desk as he drew sketches of possible surgical approaches that detailed the length of the scars. He inclined his head to the left when he discussed the pros and cons of my options at this extended visit, which my wife told me later lasted forty minutes, but which felt like two gluey hours. I tried to hear his words, but thinking of surgery, thinking of myself as someone who needed surgery, made reality feel small and deep and lonely, despite my wife's hand on my knee and Dr. A's engagement. He was energetic, crisp, lean as a lacrosse stick. He understood that even for surgeons, whose job is primarily manual, at least part of his work is conversation. But I wasn't much of a conversational partner.

My visit with Dr. Z took place a day later and was considerably briefer. His office was less comfortable, more medical;

there was no refrigerator, no sofa. There was a silver sink and a utilitarian photograph of a boat at a dock. Dr. Z was short and out of shape and wore loose blue scrubs. I felt extremely nervous, perhaps more so than I'd been with Dr. A, a little more shut down, because it was the second time that I was seeing my CT scan clipped to and illuminated by a doctor's view box. I presume he spoke; again I didn't remember a word of it when my wife questioned me afterward; I kept no list in my head of what Dr. Z looked like. I couldn't describe his face to you today. With each of these two doctors, in my impossible state of anxiety, I felt like I was watching a silent video that I played some part in.

———

There is a large body of research in social psychology about how, with limited information, we make judgments about people— about nonverbal information we collect, in a sense, with the sound off. Two decades of research studies outside of medical settings have demonstrated that viewers of soundless videos can judge with high accuracy very specific aspects of the relationship and qualities of the people in the interaction based on a mere twenty seconds of a silent clip: kinship, level of romantic involve- ment, the winner and loser of a sporting event, racial bias, per- sonality disorder, even levels of deception. Our inferences about others based on these brief glimpses or "thin slices" of nonverbal behavior are intuitive and unshakeable; they occur automatically.

These are the kinds of thin-slice judgments I must have made during my first meetings with these two surgeons. Based on body language and expression alone, I had strong impressions about certain aspects of each doctor, about his communication skills, disposition, and interpersonal manner. And it was comforting to read in the psychology literature, all these years later, that such judgments are usually quite accurate: that is, my intuitive judgment at those first visits was likely to match the judgments of other patients who'd had *extensive* personal experience with that doctor.

My wife sensibly preferred Dr. A. I chose Dr. Z. Linguist Edward Sapir characterized nonverbal behavior as "an elaborate and secret code that is written nowhere, known by none, and understood by all." Unlike conversation, the interpretation of nonverbal behavior is processed without intention, outside awareness. Even distraction has no effect on our evaluative social judgment—it happens so quickly and efficiently. Asked to count backward by seven from one thousand while watching the silent video of the interaction between two strangers, our psychological reading would not be impaired; we would continue to be accurate in judging the qualities of the actors. Sometimes we may pay attention to an idiosyncratic or vivid gesture, twitch, scratch, or hand motion, a habit we think we've smartly noticed, but our global, automatic, gestalt impressions are more powerful.

Counting backward from one thousand doesn't affect judgment, but when asked by researchers to make a list of all the possible reasons that we might like or dislike a person in a video (or a doctor in an office) just before we rate him—his stance, his stillness or jiggling, the way he opened his hands or hid his teeth when smiling, the line of his clothes, the shadow of his nose on his cheek, the hesitance of a handshake—the very act of generating and recording such a list ruins the accuracy of our judgment. This kind of brain work, this itemizing, compromises our thin-slice judgment and adversely effects our intuition.

Our perception of others actually seems to come in two distinct steps—step 1, an automatic, nonconscious part, followed by a very brief but controlled and "interpretive" step 2. These two parts occur, researchers have recognized, in seconds, but if we think of these two parts as a sequence, it's as if, at times, a cognitive logjam occurs after the initial intuitive stage of perception, slowing step 2 down, causing problems. We are slower *and* less accurate in our judgment of others if we think carefully beforehand rather than trust our step 1 "gut instinct." It seems that a careful, deliberative strategy of interpreting nonverbal cues is not only unnecessary but may actually be a hindrance. (The results are consistent when we judge based on a video, whether the sound is off or on.) Thinking and articulating, at least in regard to our initial evaluation of people, is counterproductive. There is a peril to pondering.

Before my visits, I had prepared no list of the qualities I wanted in the surgeon who would likely cut a circle through my skull and go ice fishing in my cranium. I knew that I had to make a decision relatively quickly, but other than gathering the names of two competent surgeons, I hadn't researched either of them. My decision, it turned out, was nonverbal, since I really didn't remember a word either Dr. A or Dr. Z said. The list-making I'd unknowingly done during my time with Dr. A (and hadn't done with Dr. Z because I'd already shut down by then, numb with anxiety) had doomed his chance of being my surgeon. I don't know if I was "accurate" in my automatic judgment of Dr. Z's personality, but his personality didn't matter. I would never get to know his personality. I didn't know if he was kind or compassionate; there was something more absolute driving my decision, something purged of all words, some thin slice of him that might describe my certainty. At the time, I couldn't explain my decision to my wife, who was a little shocked, a little worried about my sanity.

I now believe my choice took place before Dr. Z even spoke, and I think I can explain it, although at the time it was unconscious and instantaneous. Dr. Z moved slowly, or as I saw it, took great care in his movements. He seemed like the type of person who could sit and read on the porch on a Saturday afternoon and not feel the need to get up until the sun started to set. If it turned out that I was a late afternoon case, he wouldn't need to rush off to his tennis game. He took a long look at me when I entered his office, as if he was preparing to remark on the mass on my forehead, but he let me speak first.

I'd chosen a surgeon. Next I needed an internist who would order the required preoperative tests. I was in a different emotional state than when I'd met Dr. Z three weeks earlier. Now I was deeply, painfully sad. Going into the two consultations with prospective neurosurgeons, I'd been extremely nervous, and in fact, I'd been nervous since I'd seen the CT scan of my head and let myself dwell on the worst possible diagnoses. But after choosing my neurosurgeon, I was aware that my anxiety had transformed to sadness. I had gained the understanding that under anesthesia my life would be on the line; there were no guarantees; the surgeon could find something he wasn't expecting as he poked near my brain. I could have real trouble, even as I was anticipating a full recovery. When I looked for an internist, I was imagining life after a possibly problematic recovery.

The doctor too reads the patient nonverbally—she sees the patient's posture, his head-down stillness. A doctor's kindness is a response to a patient's sadness; the best internists detect sadness. Dr. L, the first and only internist I interviewed, did.

During our conversation she committed none of the nonverbal body-language no-no's that might have triggered an immediate, unconscious negative thin-slice judgment on my part: holding objects in front of her body; checking the time or inspecting her fingernails; picking lint off her clothes; stroking her chin while looking at me; narrowing her eyes; standing too close; looking down while listening; touching her face; resting her hands behind her head or on her hips; not directly facing me; crossing her arms; foot or finger tapping. I remember Dr. L's first words: "What can I do to help you?"

Her first words didn't drive my decision; I chose Dr. L based on the *sound* of her voice. It was the end-of-a-winter-fire kind of voice: deep, soft, moderately slow, and clearly articulated. It was anxious and concerned, almost sad. A good internist is a good worrier. Again, the research shows that we respond emotionally to a doctor's voice very powerfully and quickly, though Dr. L actually spoke very little during my visit.

Brief segments of physicians' speech patterns with patients in medical offices (audio clips lasting forty seconds) communicate unexpectedly rich information that predicts important medical outcomes, such as patient satisfaction. In these experiments, researchers filter doctors' speech from audiotaped patient-doctor interactions, eliminating the high-frequency sounds on which word recognition depends, so that only expressive features, such as intonation, speed, pitch, and rhythm, remain in these thin slices of voice; the final audiotapes include no words. Each clip is rated by a panel for warmth, concern, and dominance. The malpractice histories of the recorded doctors are known to the researchers.

The doctors whose voices are judged to be more dominant are more likely to have been sued than those who sound less dominant. There is always a power imbalance between the doctor and the patient, and patients are particularly sensitive to displays of dominance. Because the typical visit is characterized by technical explanations, there is an ever-present risk for patients to perceive that their doctor is talking down to them. In the medical encounter, "how" a message is conveyed may be as important as "what" is said. Should doctors be trained—by listening to audiotapes of their own voices at patients' first visits—to become aware of and sensitive to the manner in which they speak? Should doctors be given videos to study and improve their nonverbal behaviors? Can dominance be subtly transformed to authority?

Sadness often causes us to *over*-reason, to deliberate over our initial reaction to a stranger. Sad people don't have what William James called "effortless attention." We slow down, we deliberate over each statement we hear and every gesture we witness. This deliberation hinders the ability to make accurate judgments based only on minimal (nonverbal) information provided by the first moments of a stranger's behavior or voice. Sadness, like the silent cataloguing I'd done during my visit with Dr. A, causes a cognitive pileup after the initial intuitive stage of perception; it slows down part 2 of our thin-slice judgment, causing problems. In experiment after experiment, sad persons are less accurate and take more time than happy people to make judgments of the actors in videos.

But sadness actually affects the way we think of other people in another contradictory way. There is the immediate, silent step 2 decoding of *nonverbal* information described in the thin-slice experiments. But there is also a later, lengthier, *more* accurate step 3 coding of *verbal* information that began with the sound of Dr. L's voice and continued through the few questions she asked me: Was this my first surgery? What was I led to expect about any potential operative difficulties? How did I think she could best help me? Consumed with uncertainty and the inability to predict or control their environment, sad people (i.e., most patients thinking about their future, postoperative selves) are sensitive and careful, they listen harder and longer when interpreting social cues. Sadness is associated with heightened vigilance and increased effort in the processing of subtleties—the thoughts, feelings, and intentions of others—that come across in language.

I remember feeling that once again I was moving very slowly when I arrived at Dr. L's office. The air was viscous. In that unfortunate state, I was one of those sad people who was particularly sensitive to false reassurances and phoniness in others. I knew doctors' tricks; I used them myself. Dr. L wasn't false or phony; she admitted she hadn't seen many skull tumors. Her honesty was in keeping with her politeness.

During my worst moments of those preoperative weeks at home, I looked to my wife for reassurance and support. I looked to Dr. L for the same at this first visit. I tested her by being needy. "I'm otherwise healthy, right? So the anesthesia shouldn't be a problem?" Seeking support, I was more attuned to the display of rejection than of comfort; that day, in her cool and empty office, I felt a heightened sensitivity to unkindness. After choosing Dr. Z, I had developed a sense—as do all people with illness—that things with myself should be otherwise, that I was on unknown terrain, and that this terrain was dangerous, unsettled, tiring, and desolate. But Dr. L responded to my questions with concern, without irritation, because she understood that the sad and needy *will* demand more of a doctor's time. Sadness yields our best social accuracy when choosing those doctors whom we will spend substantial time talking to, like internists. I thought she was impressed about how calm I acted about my situation, and I wanted her to admire me. Sad people overestimate the favorable impression they make; she told me years later that I was a nervous wreck.

Meeting with a new doctor is more complicated than a lab experiment, of course. At the same time we are judging them, they are judging us. Yet my experiences as a patient fits the results of the past twenty years of thin-slice video and voice experiments. My decision about my neurosurgeon was so clearly nonreflective, automatic, nonverbal, unavailable for introspection. I was nauseously anxious to the point of deafness, the appointment akin to a silent movie. I chose an internist because I was drawn to the tone of a voice, paying attention to such details as a sad and careful listener. Happy people process information quickly and more generously, taking shortcuts, depending less on careful evaluation because it feels like it matters less. Patients are never happy to be in doctors' offices, and in a way this is good news, because they are more accurate in their judgments; with Dr. L, I judged unhappily but accurately. If things had gone wrong during Dr. Z's skull-work, I like to think Dr. L would have explained what happened, slowly, in lucid paragraphs, kindly.

As patients, we try to be responsible when searching for a new doctor. When we have the luxury of time, when it's not an emergency, we ask around. We check the national practitioner data bank for malpractice history, we look at age and training credentials, we assume that professional organizations and insurance companies have done their vetting. But the truth is that we make our selections based on little information about competence. Nor do we get to see beforehand a video clip of our doctor-to-be in action with another patient; our impressions are formed in the first minutes inside the office. Facial expressions and bows and personal distance, a smile, a lean of the body, and the tone of voice are extremely informative; they communicate information about this doctor's attitudes and feelings. At the start, we trust our personal response, and we should. We are gifted judges of the nonverbal.

There are moments when patients reveal themselves. I have to be ready. The human face and the human body are eloquent in themselves. I know, too, that as a doctor I have revealed myself in unconscious ways.

6

Random Acts of Kindness and Unkindness

It's vaguely depressing to think of
doctors as ever being unkind.

Christopher Hitchens

Friends, strangers, tell me stories about their doctor visits. They're troubled and narrate their illness story with feeling. The story is never about a physician's diagnostic acumen or procedural aptitude. It seems as though patients know exactly what kindness, or unkindness, feels like.

"My gynecologist comes into the room at my annual with a big smile. 'How nice to see you. How are things?' She remembers where I work, the names of my kids, even the name of my cat. How does she remember it all? She gives me the sense that I've been on her mind since last year. It seems that she cares, and yet it's a pure fake-out. Before she came in, I could hear her outside the door, picking up my folder, looking through it. Saying my name when she comes in gives the false impression that she knows about me. It's a trick doctors use, and I don't blame her. I know it's a trick because if she knew me so well, and had been thinking of me, why can't she read the subtext—I'm worried, I'm really not right, there's something I'm not telling her, I'm uncomfortable? This familiarity leaves us both with a problem: if she doesn't ask the right questions, I'll think she already knows about me, and I won't tell her a thing."

2.

"My fifteen-year-old daughter has torn the anterior cruciate ligament of her left knee playing basketball. She's never been in a hospital, never had surgery. I spend the night in her room, making sure she gets her pain medication, and some sleep. Her surgeon comes in at six thirty in the morning her first day post-op. He wakes her. He's a smiler, wearing blue scrubs and rubber clogs, and he has thick hair red on his forearms. When he manipulates her knee, she starts to cry with pain. When she looks away, he catches my eye and makes a sawing motion over her leg above the bad knee, pretending to chop off her leg. It quiets her, as if the limb is gone, as if this is funny in some way and we are confiding."

3.

"I went to the dermatologist last summer to have a rash on my shoulder checked. I brought my ten-year-old with me to the appointment. I remember she'd been at soccer camp that morning. I sat on the exam table, and my daughter was standing next to me reading when the doctor walked in. She greeted my daughter first, then turned to me and said, 'She has a lot of bruises. Have you had her checked for leukemia?' I thought, Are you showing me how quickly you can appraise someone who isn't even your patient? Are you demonstrating how observant you are? Or are you making a serious recommendation? Could my daughter really have leukemia? I had no interest in having her look at my shoulder after that."

4.

"'You don't want to be in the operating room any more than you need to be, and I don't want to be in the operating room any more than I need to be.' That's the kind of ambivalence I like in a doctor."

5.

"My eighty-eight-year-old father had Parkinson's disease and kept getting pneumonia. He was in and out of the hospital every month. We had stayed at the hospital late one night because he wasn't doing well. He was having a lot of trouble breathing despite the oxygen he was receiving. The doctor on call, one we'd never met before, sat my sister and me down in one of the conference rooms—the kind with a long white table covered with scraps of paper and coffee cups, next to a white board with some numbers and diagnoses on it—to discuss how to proceed, how aggressive we wanted to be with breathing treatments. He was a young man, maybe late thirties, with bags under his eyes and dark hair, and he held on to the table, trying to keep himself in his seat, trying to make us believe he wasn't in a hurry to leave. 'Eighty-eight years is a good life,' he said. Meaning, I suppose, eighty-eight years is enough. It seemed like just the wrong thing to say to us, people he didn't know. He knew nothing about my father's eighty-eight years, whether it was a good life. What if only the last few years had been good, when he'd finally reconciled with his children, and gotten to meet his grandchildren? What if he wanted a few more years to enjoy what he'd missed before?

This doctor confused age with quality. He knew nothing about my father and nothing about us."

6.

"My doctor really used to bug me asking me if I was depressed every time I came in. Until I finally got a therapist and felt much better."

7.

"When she gave me the breast biopsy result I didn't want her to say, 'We didn't find what we were hoping for. It's cancer.' I wanted to hear, 'I want you to know that you saved your own life by checking yourself. You're going to be in expert hands. There'll be a whole team of us taking care of you. You might not hear everything I have to say today because it's all so overwhelming, so I'm going to take notes for you as I go.'"

8.

"Instead of confessing his ignorance about what was causing my fever, he would burst into my room in the morning and, in this forced, cheerful voice, make pronouncements. Apparently he needed to feel that he had some news for me, when there was nothing new at all."

9.

"She touched me as if she was handling something that was delicate and precious to her. It was more than gentle; it was tender. Her touch had humility. There were no assumptions of superiority, and no sense that this was simple."

10.

"'You're overreacting,' he says to me. Would a male doctor ever say that to a man? I go to a walk-in center with neck pain and a low-grade fever. 'You just have a cold,' he says. 'You saw a tick. But you don't have a rash.' Is there any medical training that teaches young male doctors that they should never say certain things to a woman? I'm a veterinarian. I'm not afraid of ticks. I've gotten ten tick bites, and I've never had Lyme disease, but this feels different. 'Would you test me?' I ask. I almost have to beg. Would he have liked to hear me make a bigger deal about how badly I felt? I would have liked if he'd at least tried to assess if I had a good read on what was happening to me. He finally agreed to test me. When it comes back positive, I'm so angry at him, I won't speak with him on the phone. I tell his office staff where

I want the antibiotics sent. He was incompetent and unkind. Or maybe he was just lazy, making assumptions: 'Here comes another crazy woman in the summer in New England who thinks she has Lyme disease.' He had this assumption that a woman has no sense of her body."

11.

"I was with my mother-in-law in the hallway outside the ICU of this small community hospital where my father-in-law was dying. It must have been his fifth day in the hospital, and the reason for this most recent decline wasn't clear. My father-in-law had a complicated lung problem that they didn't think was pneumonia, although they weren't sure what was going on. It was about ten o'clock at night. My mother-in-law was asking the doctor on call his opinion of what had happened to her husband, what the possible causes were for his breathing trouble. Then she asked why they weren't treating him with antibiotics and what new tests were planned. All reasonable questions. When she started to ask what the options were if he got worse, the doctor said, 'I can't stand here all night talking to you, I have other patients to see.'"

12.

"The meeting lasted ninety minutes. The doctor was completely unhurried. It wasn't that he was any more encouraging than anyone else; he gave me the same cold, hard facts that the others had—basically, that my life was probably almost over. The difference was, those facts didn't seem to make him want to run away from me."

13.

"We had to put down our cat last week, and I was amazed to get a handwritten condolence card from the vet that said: 'Although saying goodbye is difficult, it is the last loving thing we can do for our cherished companions. Our thoughts are with you.' I don't know if 'jealous' is the right term, but I wish I'd gotten such a caring letter from a doctor when my first husband died."

14.

"I had an EMG a few years earlier, trying to diagnose the cause of the neuropathy in my legs. The test involves placing needles at various points along my leg and sending electric currents through them. The doctor knows I've had the test before; he has it in his records. He must have written down how painful it was for me, how much I hated it. Or at least he should have recorded how many times I'd turned down his request to do it again. When I final agree to repeat the EMG to check on the progress of my condition, I'm lying on the exam table in his office in a sweat. He starts putting in his needles and I wince. After a few more needles, I groan. 'Stop being a baby,' he says, smiling, as if this is encouragement or will make it hurt less. It only means he won't have to think about how he's hurting me. I'm so angry I don't say anything. I shut down. I want to scream, 'Have you had this test? Let's see if you're a baby when someone does it to you!'"

15.

"The best gift a doctor every gave me? At my first visit to his office after my heart attack, I told my doctor I'd been dreaming of omelets. He wrote me a prescription for a weekly omelet and handed it to my wife."

16.

"He says, 'We'll have you admitted on Monday. We only admit emergencies on weekends.' I say, 'Acute leukemia's not an emergency?' He says, 'You should relax this weekend. But come to the emergency room if you start bleeding.'"

17.

"When you get sick you find out that there's a lot of information out there. Before this visit, no doctor ever offered to find an article or research paper for me. When she went into her office and printed something out for me, that meant a lot."

18.

"I take my thirteen-year-old son to the emergency room with a foot laceration. The doctor, whom he doesn't know, sees that he has Type 1 diabetes. She tells my son that he needs to take good care of himself, that he's at risk for blindness and heart disease and kidney failure. She tries to scare him and I explode: 'How dare you presume that my son doesn't take care of himself or know anything about diabetes?'"

19.

"The doctor says to me, 'How does your husband feel about these ten extra pounds?'"

20.

"The doctor said, 'Of all the cancers you can get, this is the best.' Was he just unconscious of how it sounded? 'Best' is not the best word, I told him."

7

Lying

When regard for truth has been broken down or even
slightly weakened, all things will remain doubtful.

St. Augustine

Patrick arrives at my office complaining of back pain and reports
falling from a ladder. He's twenty-four and he looks vaguely familiar, with his long, damp brown hair under a baseball cap. Wearing a thin winter coat, he has rock-salt gray teeth and black jeans.
I find, when I search my electronic medical record system, that
we'd met four months earlier. He'd been referred to me by the
emergency room staff because he needed a primary care doctor.
He'd been treated in the ER three days before for a broken wrist,
and they'd put his injured arm in a plastic cast from his palm to
his mid-forearm. At that visit I did a full physical exam, which
was normal other than his casted right arm, and had prescribed

him sixteen Vicodin because his wrist was still "throbbing" and he wouldn't be seeing his orthopedist for another few weeks.

Patrick's cast is now gone, but his back is "killing" him. On this April morning the new buds make the trees outside my window look blurry.

"I was cleaning the snow from a customer's carport gutter, and I slipped." He tells me he does handyman work with a friend, maybe twenty hours a week. As he talks, Patrick keeps his hat on and his eyes down, in deference or evasion. During the exam, I ask him to lie on his back on my examining table and lift his left leg; he moans and winces. I begin to lift his other leg—I've barely moved him—and he quickly moans again, but louder. It's unusual for patients to experience equal pain in both legs at exactly the same angle of elevation. I ask him to stand up beside the table and try to touch his toes. He can't touch his toes, but it seems like he's hardly trying. This second visit to me in four months for a complaint that might require a pain pill prescription, and the perfect timing of his moan, make me suspicious that he wants more Vicodin. I put my hand on the middle of Patrick's spine and gently push him toward his untied sneakers. He curls a little more; his reaction, his next moan, is delayed. If the pain were severe, he would have called out for me to stop after the slightest movement. I've got him; I know he's lying. I know what he's come for.

Why doesn't his lying bother me?

"When I examine your back, I don't find any major problems. No broken bones, no torn ligaments, no herniated discs. But you're in pain," I say. "So how do you think I can best help you?" I can't know if he's truly experiencing pain—but I don't want to announce my doubt yet; I don't want to take his reason for coming away from him.

When I was a young doctor, it was troubling when a patient tried to dupe me, even more troubling when I actually was duped. I felt disrespected—not as clever as I thought I was. Being lied to felt like being pushed in the back, my authority knocked off balance. More than that, patients' lying put me at risk of missing a life-threatening diagnosis. When patients lied they were preventing me from doing my job. Slowly, I came to understand that what every patient tells me is never completely accurate, even if they have no desire to misrepresent their symptoms. They don't remember exactly when their problem started. Was it before or after the intercontinental flight? They're poor judges of duration. Did the chest pain last seconds or minutes? They fill in blanks; they try to convey what they mean. They search for a plot made up of symptoms—causation, reaction, decision, sequence—that makes illness more intelligible than it really is. They rearrange symptoms to tell a coherent explanatory narrative, which can't be the way the problem actually unfolded. They swear it happened one way, but it didn't. There's a final version only after multiple retellings and clarifications and questions—yes, they did take antibiotics last month; yes, they have been taking ibuprofen for days, come to think of it; no, the rash came before the cough. Every patient is an unreliable narrator. But inaccuracy is different from lying. The moral question is whether a patient intends to mislead. Patrick intended to mislead.

Lying breaks the social bond. Lying abrades the human connection. Lying is a refusal of connection. Substitute "addiction" for "lying" in those three sentences and you begin to see how addiction and lying are related. I have come to expect persons who misuse drugs to mislead, to lie. Patrick is lying and I'm quite sure that Patrick is addicted to opioids.

When you watch intervention shows on TV, you hear about addicts "in denial," as if it's the name of a disease. Lying is a symptom of denial. If I understand that lying is *the* symptom of addiction, then it follows that I should allow people with addictions to be exceptions to a general medical policy against lying, in the same way that I'm tolerant of an anxious person's irritability or bad temper. I understand that most doctors have no patience for people with addictions because they feel they have little time to spare— diagnosing and then dealing with a lie takes time, backtracking through an addict's disregard for the truth. I relate to people who misuse drugs the way I relate to all patients—with curiosity, compassion, and distrust in their reliability. Only the proportion of these differs depending on the patient. Given what I've learned over the years about addiction, I don't have the same reflexive cynicism as many doctors do when an addicted person lies.

"You think I'm fine? Without even an X-ray?" Patrick asks. When he takes off his cap, I see he has a long, angular face, lines on his forehead like a worried child. "My back is messed up." Sitting in the chair beside my desk, he glares at me with parted lips and an air of despair.

Should I tell him what I suspect? The requirement that physicians be honest with patients is absent from every medical oath and code of ethics. There is no discussion in medical school about when or when not to tell the truth. Because there is no official guidance as to when deception may be justified, it's simplest if doctors insist on honesty at all times: we must not lie to dying patients (even if it mitigates fear); we ridicule placebos—although they may have power—because as a rule we do not deceive. We know that patients can be injured or lose trust if they learn they have been misled.

Therefore (the logic goes), if we are honest with patients, they should be honest with us. We may even believe we have a gift for seeing not only patients' transparency but also their inclination toward the truth, no matter how they fidget or dodge or defend themselves. Truth can be recognized, but if I were to say that all addicted persons lie, I would be at risk of being too sure and omniscient.

I've heard that "there's no truth in addiction, just each addict's experience." That's one of the lies. Because there *is* truth, universally recognizable to persons addicted to drugs. Here it is: *My drug was the greatest thing ever, the first time, and for a while.* Here it is: *It was unmanageable from the start.* Here it is: *It caused more trouble than I thought it would.* Here it is: *Things will get worse.* These are truths.

Conversations in my office are always coercive, always one-sided. There is an expectation that I can ask anything, and if answered honestly, I will do my best to provide a remedy. The doctor asks a question and the patient never says, "Why do you ask?"—unless the patient has something to hide. A lie can be an evasion of self-awareness or a way to sustain a story or a way to smooth things over.

Interview thirty people with addictions and there's a standard list of lies. I didn't sit behind a dumpster to use, I didn't sell my body, I didn't fall down at the wedding, or forget to lock the door, or fall asleep at work, or leave the stove on. I do what everyone else does. I don't act differently. If something bad happens, even if there is evidence, there's nothing wrong with me.

They lie once, a little lie. Then they lie again. And again. At a certain point, they can't go back.

Maybe Patrick believes I can't tell he's lying. Maybe he's looking for sympathy. Maybe he can't tell a true story anymore. Maybe he doesn't lie on purpose, he's just accustomed to making shit up.

"Here's the thing," I say to Patrick. I speak slowly, because there's no better way to spook an addict than by talking too fast. "I don't know if you fell off a ladder or not, but I don't really believe that your back hurts that much."

Earlier in my career, I would never have said such a thing. I would have ducked the possibility of conflict. I knew that people with drug problems would get angry when I doubted them. Together we would have to do a song and dance around the truth. I knew they would say, "I have no idea what you're talking about." But with Patrick today, none of this bothers me, because I keep in mind that parsing lies is part of my job. I remind myself: addicts are lying when their lips are moving. I want to see that we get to a different kind of visit, where perhaps I can offer latitude, forgiveness, to someone obviously in desperate straits. Lies are enslaving; addiction is enslaving.

Patrick's expression suddenly changes. "If I don't tell you the truth, how can you help me get better?" he asks with false innocence, as though now that he's caught him in the lie, he has decided that a doctor's office can change a person's way of being. He lies about lying. He *hadn't* told me the truth at first, and there was no evidence he wanted to *get better* in the sense of stopping his drug use. "I need a Vicodin script," he says.

"Tell me why."

Doctors and patients don't have the usual social bond. The patient comes in with symptoms; my job is to relieve those symptoms. That's the bond. The connection is transactional: Patrick needs a prescription today. Sometimes a prescription for pain medication will save an addict some cash, or a street hustle. For most addicts, the ideal appointment would be a prescription slid under the door, and the absence of me and my questions. That way no one can tell them that they don't need what they claim to need.

"I had to lie to the policeman who searched me today after I ran a stop sign," Patrick says. By "had to" he means it seemed reasonable for him to lie. "I was able to pass the walk-a-straight-line test, but I lied when the cop found pills in my pocket. I knew it was illegal to have those pills, so I said I had a prescription, I just didn't have the prescription bottle with me. I told him it was at home. He could have hauled me in, but I knew this cop's brother from high school, and the cop told me to bring the little plastic container down to the station as proof later in the day. So I came back to see you."

He smiles, proud of his explanation. Patrick wants to avoid a possession charge. He needs pills, and a pill bottle with my name on it, and his name, and the name of a narcotic. Not only as proof for the police that he doesn't make his living buying and selling loose pills, but also as a means to prevent opioid withdrawal, which will arrive soon now that he is out of pills. My prescription would solve both of his immediate problems. But his request asks me to join in on his lie.

"I have to admit that I'm not a very good liar," Patrick says.

"No, you're not," I say, but with respect for his new state of self-knowledge and sincerity.

"Years of dishonesty and I have very little to show for it."

Is that true? Addicts deploy lies not only to convince me of their innocence, but also in the service of completing a story that explains them to me. When I ask questions, chances are they know how to answer because they've been asked before. Addiction makes them inventive ("I fell from a ladder") and forces them to keep secrets. People with addictions know more about what they want than they let on. They don't trust anyone, so they think, "He'd have to be a fool to trust me. What does it matter if what I'm looking for here in his office doesn't work out? There are other doctors."

I have learned from my practice that if knowledge is power, then every visit to a doctor makes a patient feel powerless. Lies redistribute power; they advantage the liar, disadvantage the deceived. Manipulation provides a feeling of ascendancy, of escape from powerlessness.

"I'd like to hear about those years of dishonesty," I say to Patrick. "I'm interested."

I want to turn what seems a rare occasion of honesty from Patrick into a way to learn more about his addiction. I have already forgiven him for his initial back pain lie. I thought about a cold February day years before when a woman had brought her twenty-year-old daughter in to see me. The daughter lived in the basement apartment the mother had let her fix up, and she'd been vomiting for almost two days. She had all the typical flu symptoms: a headache, a runny nose, muscle aches. She couldn't sleep. Her fever was down from the Tylenol. Still, her mother was worried; she was convinced it was bad seafood from the group home where her daughter worked as an aide. She'd had to drag her daughter into my office. I gave this worried mother a list of possibilities, most of them infectious. She became more concerned when she heard that hepatitis was on the list.

When I asked her mother to leave the room during the examination, the daughter looked down at my shoes and told me she'd run out of Perc 30's three days earlier. Nothing contagious about that. When I learned the truth, I felt bad for her, for the pain she was in now and the sorrow ahead. And I knew I would feel bad when I lied to her mother, when this patient made me into a liar too.

That day I began to understand that some patients have to lie. They were mostly beaten-down women and men, trying to do good, unable to quell their own distress in any useful way. They became criminal or cruel as a means of outmaneuvering their circumstances. They lied about little stuff and big stuff. For people who feel their lives are insignificant, or a mess, perhaps lying is not really a vexing dilemma. It may seem like the best alternative, like self-defense, like survival. The worst addicts are the worst liars.

"When I got here today, I thought I might as well lie to you," Patrick admits. "I thought you wouldn't believe me anyway if I told you the truth." In other words: I can never persuade anyone of anything. Feel free to doubt me. It's a twisted request for understanding, or a clever, disorienting ruse. Patrick embodies a strange quality that is inherent in addicts: the fake sounds exactly the same as the real.

He gives me a weary smile, as though he knows that between him and anyone he speaks to, there is none of the trust that sustains most ordinary conversation. Sometimes people with addictions come from families with a long tradition of suffering. Still, their families—stolen from, threatened, yelled at, lied to—can't stand them. You know you're an addict when no one can bear you. No one can stand addicts, except other addicts (and the odd doctor), and then only if they provide the substance itself or a safe place to use it.

I wonder if Patrick believes we've made an implicit deal here: if he's honest with me, I'll give him the prescription he came for.

I don't have an all-absorbing preoccupation with truth, which perhaps makes it easier for me to come to grips with the deception of people with addictions. Reasons to lie occur to most people quite often—lies can be helpful, useful, a necessity. Many lies are trivial. I've lied to save face, to protect others, to avoid a fight. I lie when I don't pick up the phone, pretending not to be available.

To condemn Patrick is unnecessary. He lies from shame, to erase shame, to protect himself, although he injures himself in the process. The risk of a patient lying all the time is that when my help is actually wanted, I may be unable to distinguish truthful messages from deceptive ones.

"I guess you see a lot of patients with addictions," Patrick says. "Were you an addict?" he asks hopefully. Other patients have asked. They ask when they come to the point where they believe they will never be understood except by other addicts. I could lie. For some, it would be helpful if I had been an addict; they would believe I wouldn't judge them.

"I am not an expert in addiction," I say, "but in getting out of addiction."

I try never to say, "I understand your addiction." The more introspective addicts realize that even *they* don't quite understand what happened to them over the past decade, how they ended up in my office. The medications I offer to treat their addiction are not meant to help them understand themselves. The goal is to free them of the desire for that drug. Those aims could be complementary, but it is the second that allows the first.

I ask Patrick to tell me the last time he was dishonest with a doctor. He tells me about a time a few months ago when he read up on the symptoms of a migraine before he went to an emergency room. There he told them he was allergic to Tylenol. He said ibuprofen hadn't worked at home. Even when he got only one dose of something strong, that was something. A small victory. Then he got a prescription for ten pills—a greater success. Then he tells me about the ER visit before that one when he went in complaining of shoulder pain. And the time before that it was cancer he said was being treated out of state. A few times he'd checked into detox for a day. A vacation from the shelter. Three squares and a bed with only one roommate. He stepped out for a cigarette break and never came back. He tells me he has to remember the places he's been and the lies he's told so he's able to repeat them.

He offers this history as though he doesn't even know the man he's describing; he tells it without emotion. It was from another life, somewhere else.

He thinks of himself as an expert in falsehood. Lying is tried and true. Or, better: tried and not true. Lying emerges as a daily, hourly occurrence for Patrick. As with all people in need, he probably feels threatened and suspicious most of the time; he fears a trap. He must be careful—each lie has to be perfect. He has to keep an absolute and uncompromising allegiance to the untrue.

Why should I be judgmental? It would deprive Patrick of one of the instruments for getting better: me. If I free him of desire for his addictive love, he can stop the lies he uses in order to satisfy that desire.

Patrick is on a roll. He checks my eyes to see if I want him to continue. I can see he is enthusiastic and adept, a salesman. Gregarious, funny, almost manic now. Has his drug withdrawal induced this behavior or revealed his true character? He sells stories. Maybe that's why I like him—he does what I do in my writing life. Does lying make you a sociopath or a better story-teller? There are lots of ways to sell. The truth is singular and lies are plural. He laughs and exaggerates. He wants to make a strong impression. Memorable salesmen always have a danger-ous energy. At the same time, he gives off an aura that makes me believe he wants to please me. He needs to have passion and also be credible. He knows he needs not to appear misleading.

He is selling me on the possibility that he will not lie to me again. He is trying to make me buy that I am his last best hope. If he is lying, he is lying optimistically.

I'm not going to lie: I have a grudging respect for the skill and craft of Patrick's wordplay and pain in the back act. Instead of being disappointed or disapproving, I'm mildly amused. I don't feel the sting of having been deceived.

Patrick turns back to today's police story. "I don't want to go to jail," he says.

I know he doesn't want to go jail because a cop found a pill in his pocket. But I know he has other ready defenses for lying. *Who does it harm if I want to get high anyway?* Another is, *I can't help myself. Addiction is an altered state. Do you hold the person who talks in his sleep responsible for what he says?* Another is, *If I don't get you to prescribe to me, I will go into terrible withdrawal and will be in crisis, and I might have to rob to get what I need. So isn't lying the less evil?* As if this utilitarian justification would remove moral blame.

When I want the truth, I ask for a photograph. Patrick takes out his phone, hesitates. I ask for a picture from when he was younger, from before he started using. He shows me a grandmother he's cooking with in a kitchen somewhere. He is a good-looking teenager, hair to his shoulders, gleaming teeth. He shows me pictures of himself and a series of beautiful dogs. Photos can lie, of course, but not in this case. The last few years have aged him.

As a physician, I need someone to root for. I root for Patrick's other identities, the ones he doesn't lie about: best dog groomer, caring grandson, keeper of the perfect lasagna recipe. The truth stopped when he got to the one identity—addict—that makes all of the others irrelevant.

I want my patients' secrets. To not know them is to miss their life. Maybe that's why I can wait out their lies and easy duplicity, their casual withholding of information. I can ask them to retell, but I have to find the right tone when I doubt their story.

Addicted persons live between wishes—to feel better, to use more without consequences, to make sure no one finds out. The admission of addiction is more painful than quitting altogether. Patrick's truthfulness—about his fear of jail, about his years of dishonesty—surprises me. Like an apology, it takes me aback. I'm grateful. I try hard. To practice medicine is to develop loyalty to certain abstractions: wellness, self-care, prevention of premature death, longevity. Shouldn't truth be on this list?

There was something Patrick believed would satisfy him and in the most fundamental sense wanted, or believed he wanted, that opioids could provide, but in the pursuit, he's destroying himself. If Patrick can tell the truth to one person, if he can say to himself—and, better yet, out loud—that he's had the wrong picture of satisfaction, it will be the beginning of a transformation.

Maybe this honesty is the beginning. But today he needs a prescription. I write it, the prescription for the medication he's named. I give him four tablets as a gesture of goodwill so he'll come back to see me. If he returns, I plan to ask him what I ask every addict with whom I'm just getting acquainted: What kind of person do you want to be? If a patient answers, "Anything other than an addict," I'm optimistic. This answer means: I will no longer have to lie about who I am. The aim of addiction treatment is to get to this answer, this redescription.

When Patrick returns a week later, I'm hopeful. When he sees me staring at his pinpoint pupils, he tells me the light in my room is too bright. When I ask for details about his visit to the police station, he seems surprised, which means whatever he's about to say next will be unpleasant, unverifiable, untruthful. He's not in jail. I don't even know if the police story was true.

He asks for a few more Vicodin, as though we've reached a new level of understanding and agreement. When I ask, "What kind of person do you want to be?" he says, "It's complicated," and I know I won't be able to help Patrick today.

8

Accidental Kindness

One of the things that makes kindness in doctoring tricky is that kindness is in the eye of the beholder: what feels kind to one patient could feel cruel to another.

Some patients do not do well when given options; to them, clear instruction can be a form of kindness, and the doctors who offer it are appreciated as competent and confident. Other patients want to know about as many alternatives as possible, even ones the doctor himself might not recommend or choose. Practicing kindness often depends on the careful, unpredictable work of ascertaining which kind of patient you're dealing with.

That was the challenge when Mrs. Narayan walked into my small exam room, a woman in her seventies with gray-streaked black hair to her waist, slowly leading a younger man who appeared to be her son. She was wearing a beautiful sari—red, purple, and yellow—and sandals. He was wearing a suit, a pressed white shirt with a stiff collar that edged into his neck, and black shoes that were brilliantly shined. They sat side by side with identical postures on my simple metal chairs. I placed myself in from of them on a rolling stool. He introduced himself as Amit Narayan.

"Let me tell you. My mother is not like this. This is not how she is all of her life since she moved here two years ago. It has not been good for a month now. She is not acting herself. You must find a satisfactory way to help her. I can translate if necessary."

This was not the way most visits started in my office, with such urgency, or with an interlocutor. He was a small man who looked to be in his midthirties. His nails were manicured, his watch elegant. His feet tapped, agitated next to her calm. She kept her hands folded on her lap, fingers knit directly below her kamarband. Her eyes opened and closed very slowly.

"She no longer cooks, or doesn't have an interest when she does. When shopping, she is distracted. My mother cooks without her normal preparation; she will not peel, she asks my wife to chop for her, she makes lentils without salt and also without a smile. It is a change in behavior. She is depressed in many ways, my wife says."

He stopped to speak in his own language to her and Mrs. Narayan answered him in English so that I understood.

"I am not depressed," she said, "I am afraid."

As an internist working in a private office, I was scheduled to spend thirty minutes with Mrs. Narayan and her son. As a new patient, she received a "double slot," twice the length of a standard fifteen-minute follow-up visit. I had twenty-eight slots between 8 A.M. and 4 P.M., four per hour for seven hours with an hour for lunch (usually a time to finish writing my electronic chart notes from the morning). I often found my schedule over-booked as the day moved along, that is, two patients would be scheduled for the same time slot, and I sometimes ended up seeing thirty-two patients in a day as I had made it a rule never to turn away patients who were suddenly ill and wanted an appointment. If I did not make room for them, their choice was to wait a day or go to an emergency room or walk-in clinic where they would see someone they didn't know.

My staff, however, did not like this double-booking. When I was double-booked the waiting area became overcrowded (I shared my waiting room with other doctors), and there was more work for the secretaries and medical aides who ran the place—each extra patient generated another intake check of address and insurance, room assignment, vital signs and weight, test ordering, vaccine or EKG administration, billing, and follow-up appointment planning—on top of the endless phone calls, medication refills, scanning of documents and reports into patient records, and reminder letters the office staff was processing. Our office generally ran smoothly and happily. As in any small work space, there were jointly signed, gently teasing birthday cards, takeout Chinese lunches, and sharing of phone photos and gossip and resentment—a sense, when certain dyads or triads could speak frankly in the break room, that *certain people* were not doing their fair share of the day's work.

Although her son started off the conversation, I wanted to hear from Mrs. Narayan. But for the moment, this was not to be.

"The cardiologist has frightened her," Amit Narayan said.

"She's seen a cardiologist recently?" I asked.

"Her heart attack. You've not heard this, then? I asked for the records to be sent to you when they arranged this appointment as she was leaving the hospital." It was as if he was already irritated, or his anger had continued unabated since her cardiology visit.

"When was this?"

"A month ago." She had slighter darker skin than her son. They had similar coffee-dark eyes, slim noses.

"No, I haven't gotten any records yet. Sometimes these things are slow."

"In the age of computers, information transfer should not be slow. I am in the technology business. There is no good reason for these results not to have arrived once we signed for the transfer."

Of course he was right—although the hospital's electronic health record system and the one used by my office were not the same, so hospital documents had to be faxed or mailed to me—but I didn't want to agree. That would have seemed like an admission of wrongdoing and an indication that he should continue talking. I really wanted to hear from her.

"The cardiologist believes she is best served by a general doctor at this time as she awaits her next procedure. So we are here, although I'm not sure of your function."

"I suppose your cardiologist believes I can help your mother comfortably wait, or maybe I can add a different point of view." I turned to my patient. "Have you had any chest pain since leaving the hospital?"

"She knows to report it, and she has reported none," Amit said.

There were cultural and generational reasons why children spoke for their parents. There were language barriers and severe cognitive problems that forced a child to step in. I wanted to interrupt him to ascertain if any of these applied to his mother, or if he was just a man speaking for a woman he believes he is protecting but may actually be misrepresenting. His face had no wrinkles, like his mother's.

"I tell her not to be afraid," Amit said, "but I know that what she fears is that she will die. I tell her that she is not about to die, she looks as well as ever, even if the doctor suggests surgery."

I could sense that Amit Narayan had great expectations of his mother's cardiologist, although he also disapproved of his information transfer skills, and perhaps even of this referral to me. Many patients, and their children, still held the expectations of the antibiotic era, the greatest success of twentieth-century medicine, the treatment of infectious disease: they believe that doctors can cure. Yet the antibiotic precedent barely applied to the twenty-first-century patient, with her list of chronic diseases that so often included heart disease. The public misunderstanding of modern medicine was only made worse by the dye-injecting catheterizations, the CT, MRI, and PET scans that provided seemingly unerring images of the previously unseen, pointing doctors to what needed fixing. Because the public expected that every disease could be found and fixed, it expected that there was a remedy with a prescription or procedure for every major cause of illness. There were corrections for every problem—stents for coronary disease, neurotransmitter adjusters to sharpen cognition, gene-based therapies to individualize chemotherapies, immune modulators for inflammatory conditions, seven-day diets, erectile agents so potent they may last *too* long, pain pills that were fully effective without making us sleepy or constipated or addicted. The public learned of these marvels via direct-to-patient advertising, driving the cultural expectation of immediate, simplistic, and unrealistic solutions.

So my patients often felt disappointed. A patient could easily feel resentful as her body was betraying her, when she was terrified, when she realized she didn't *have* a body but *was* her body, when she felt alone, a feeling that all illness induced. This resentment would inevitably be directed at doctors, at me. Mrs. Narayan's son was already a bit disappointed in the cardiologist who scared his mother, or at least didn't assuage her fear, and then didn't even get the information to my office in time for her visit. Although he was also prepared to take this same expert's advice, I could tell that Amit Narayan was important and disapproving when he was at work. As his employee, you'd think, at first glance, he was pleasant enough, but he wasn't, the way tea unexpectedly dries your mouth. I immediately sensed that he expected my "general doctor" care to be unsatisfactory as well.

"Here is his card," Amit said, withdrawing Dr. Humphreys's info from his wallet. "I am sure he will tell you what his best plan is." He said this as if he didn't think much of Humphreys himself, while believing that the cardiologist's plan was obviously the one to follow.

I knew Dr. William Humphreys pretty well. He listened with his head tilted. Humphreys was one of those doctors who wore indifference as a mask. He had protective layers, but also depth of feeling. He believed the universe was a horror show, and he wanted to do something about it. He accepted no whining, no slacking, no life-is-futile self-pity from doctor or patient. You would never hear Bill Humphreys say, "It doesn't matter," about any subject. Everything mattered. Working to get a patient some relief was his way of being empathetic.

"Practicing cardiology," Humphreys once explained to me, "is the opposite of gambling. Instead of the pleasure of a little loss, a little profit, you have to win every time." What I understood him to be saying was "Gamblers are cheerful people, they're optimists, but doctors have to be cautious because we're betting on every man and woman." When he was right about something, Humphreys made a polite attempt to conceal his simple, serious satisfaction.

Humphreys's need to control life, call the shots, do it his way, was another way of controlling his patients' destinies. He expected others to yield to his will. He told people when to have tests, when to return for a visit, when they needed a procedure. He had secure beliefs that he offered to patients who were fearful in the insecure world of illness. Nothing astonished him or caused difficulties. His red hair glistened in the artificial light. He was the kind of doctor that everyone liked.

I stepped out of the office holding the card Amit had given me, and reached Humphreys on the phone. Mrs. Narayan had *not* had a heart attack, it turned out. She had been hospitalized with unstable angina and was *at risk* for a heart attack; her symptoms had been controlled with three medications before she left the hospital. There had been no damage to her heart. He had recommended surgery to deal definitively with her coronary blockages. I didn't ask whether he'd told her that she was at imminent risk of dying, as her son said she feared.

On hanging up with Humphreys, I decided I would correct her son's misinformation and review with Mrs. Narayan the facts of her heart disease and potential treatment options, as she understood them—both the threat of demise and the chance of survival—when I returned to the room.

Mrs. Narayan was very still in her seat and her son was standing with his back to her, staring out the window that overlooked the parking lots where steamrollers were flattening new areas to be paved.

"I spoke to Dr. Humphreys. He told me that you didn't have a heart attack and that your catheterization showed three blockages that should be dealt with sooner or later."

Even though she had had a heart catheterization that had outlined her arterial blockages, Mrs. Narayan was dealing, in some ways, with an abstraction. She did not see her illness, did not touch it. She didn't know the color or the texture of coronary plaque. Humphreys might have shown her the scan's shadows, the fuzzy X-ray of her three blocked arteries, but like most patients' problems, hers were protected by skin and muscle and rib, underground, unopened.

"But that is not what he said to us," said her son. "He said that there is no *later*. If this is not taken care of, she will die."

Accidental Kindness

Had Humphreys tried to scare her? Fear had made her stop chopping onions and forced her son to drive her to my office.

"Did Dr. Humphreys explain the procedure he thought it best to perform?"

Cardiologists, all specialists who focus on chronic conditions like heart disease, were trained to be contemptuous (suspicious) of patients feeling well, and Mrs. Narayan was not in distress. As if it was fraudulent, covering up an underlying problem. Or as if patients could too easily fall for transient good news when something awful was on the way. Lab reports and scans offered the truer, hidden, narrative: you will soon be overtaken. The discourse about health was driven by dire warnings and extreme advice. When patients lived in fear, they followed advice. It was something to do in defense against pending disaster. The secret, bodily narrative was sinister; the way forward was simple and clear.

"He said that my mother would be best served by open heart surgery. Is there some question you have about his plan?" Amit asked.

"What do you think of this plan?" I asked her. I wanted to understand how she interpreted what Humphreys had advised, but Amit monopolized the conversation.

Some patients were weighed down by a sense of incomprehension; they left my office feeling ignorant because I hadn't explained myself well, or because the terrified mind distorts what it learns. This sense that a visit had sped up, that what they thought they'd heard may not be what was meant, left patients frustrated and scared, and I presumed that this had happened during the hospitalization when Mrs. Narayan had met Bill Humphreys. Sometimes the idea of illness arrived too quickly to incorporate; patients were not ready to learn the truth about their bodies. Looking ahead, patients sometimes could not get to the next decision, blocked by the fear of worst outcomes. Sometimes the decisions patients were asked to make were too large; they asked their grown children to make them.

Amit interrupted. "My mother was a mathematics professor. She is a very intelligent woman. But my mother of course doesn't want this bypass surgery. She also is not ready to die."

Her son was scared, but I didn't know about Mrs. Narayan.

"Did the cardiologist *tell* you that you were about to die?" I asked, looking directly at Mrs. Narayan.

"He said I am at risk," she said. Her voice was neither nervous nor overcautious.

"You know of course that *everyone* with coronary disease is at risk." I watched her watching me, trying to read my face.

"Then you agree with his opinion," Amit said.

Once someone had brought up the possibility of dying, it was difficult to turn the conversation elsewhere for very long. In most patient conversations at the start of what I knew would become a chronic illness—the treatment of low back pain or debilitating arthritis of the knee—I was able to find alibis to sidestep certain prognoses and sure answers; I could find respite from a difficult discussion. My view had always been that medicine put together a rigidly simple account of illness. Based on notions of objectivity, medicine took its tone of truth from science. In my own life, I resisted the idea that medicine offered a single answer or could predict a single outcome. I projected this resistance onto Mrs. Narayan. In my office, I functioned in a state of low-level skepticism, which was also a state of acute focus. I didn't mean to be anti-Humphreys and aimless; after a career of aiming, my mind constantly ran lists of options. With chronic problems that were incurable, I wasn't necessarily sure what to recommend. Long ago I'd convinced myself that with patients, the essence of judgment was knowing when, or if, to exercise my ignorance.

"Your lungs sound clear. Your heart rhythm is steady," I said to her during the examination. She sat on the exam table, and without asking her to undress, I worked my stethoscope under her sari. A more thorough exam was unnecessary, as she had been in the hospital not long before and been examined many times. Her son remained in the room. "Dr. Humphreys told me that your heart has incurred no damage. The heart muscle is strong, normal." What I heard through the stethoscope was a question she hadn't yet asked. I thought of a question I would have wanted to be asked in her position.

"No one wants bypass surgery," I said. "If you weren't *at risk*, as your cardiologist put it, what would you plan to do in the next month?"

"I would go to India," she said without pausing. "I would go to India to see my sister who is dying."

"But she cannot go," her son said, annoyed that she had even brought up this far-fetched idea. "Due to her heart condition."

"Who says she can't go?" I asked. I was trying to be provocative. I was speaking for her, this mathematician who had spoken barely at all. I was speaking for her against the idea that a doctor's recommendation must always be faced and accepted, even or especially at the cost of those very things that we most desire. Such rote acceptance disallowed imagination, which had its own power and ferocity and health.

"Her cardiologist wanted her to prepare for surgery immediately," Amit said. It seemed that Bill Humphreys's presentation had been straightforward, and Amit Narayan had heard the advice, but perhaps his mother had other ideas and would make up her own mind.

"That's his job," I said to the two of them. "To tell you how to fix the problem you have. But if you plan to have surgery, when to have it? That is your job to decide."

Her son was shaking his head in disagreement. "How can she go?"

"She can go if she knows and understands the risk and she chooses to go. She may choose not to go.

"I don't know if you came here for my opinion, but that is my opinion." I had not been casual in offering my provocation.

"What is my mother's risk in your opinion?" Amit asked.

"She has blockages, but she is not in pain. She walked into my office today; they let her go home from the hospital. If she needed emergency surgery, Dr. Humphreys would have kept her. She will take the medications Dr. Humphreys has already prescribed. There is probably a very slightly higher risk during the flights, but we can talk to the cardiologist to find out if she needs oxygen or something more. There will be the upset and joy of seeing her sister. She will have nitroglycerin if she needs it. There are hospitals in India."

"She could die if she goes."

"She could die if she stays," I said. "Even if the risk is slightly higher if you travel, to my mind it's not unreasonable if you decide to go," I said to Mrs. Narayan, before turning back to Amit. "People take risks all the time to do what they value doing. She can have surgery when she returns."

He began to object, but she grabbed his wrist, the six golden bracelets on her own wrist sliding toward her tightening fingers. Her eyes did not let go of mine.

"I am not afraid to die," she said. "My son has misunderstood. When I say that I am afraid, it is that I will not have the chance to see my sister before she dies.

"This is a kindness," she said. She smiled for the first time. She breathed deeply with her clear lungs. I felt a nerve-end tremulousness that I had gotten it right.

9

Forgiveness

PART I

When I heard that the surgeon and the patient he'd injured during an operation and left disfigured were willing to speak to me, I was surprised and, more than anything, relieved. I'd recently made my mistake with Beatriz. Still shaken from that incident, in short order I made two other, far smaller, errors in judgment with longtime patients—a poor choice of medication prescription that caused a dangerous fall in blood sugar in one man, a delay in answering a phone call that sent an older woman unnecessarily to the emergency room in the other. Neither was irreversible, but both patients were now angry with me, maybe irreparably. Every act of incompetence I committed after Beatriz made me think of her, a patient who'd never returned to my practice and made me feel unkind, not careful enough. Every error also made me think of my father and his doctor, who I had always believed malpracticed and caused my father's death.

Troubled by my ineptitude that month and the fact that neither Beatriz nor my other patients would take my calls when I tried to reach them to apologize, puzzled and feeling guilty, I'd taken time out of work, trying to understand what I'd done and how I'd bungled the care of my patients. I wanted to get back to work, but without the whirring in my brain. I was hoping that by talking to the surgeon and his patient I might think of my office as a less depressing place and find pleasure again in the work I loved.

I'd asked a mutual friend to introduce me to each of them so I could hear their stories for myself. According to my friend, somehow, at this point two years after the surgery, the patient bore no ill will toward the surgeon. I emailed the surgeon and his patient and told them I was a writer and a doctor interested in how doctors and patients overcome medical mistakes and in this case how they had come to accept each other. While they might have reached some tentative level of understanding, what had she done with her anger and he with his guilt? This patient (I'll call her Ms. P) could yet decide to bring a malpractice suit against him (I will call him Dr. S) as a kind of punishment for the facial damage she had suffered; he would have to live with the ongoing anxiety of that prospect.

Did Dr. S deserve punishment even if he'd done nothing out of the ordinary and something had gone unfortunately, operatively wrong? The lawsuit, if there ever were to be one, would be a staging area for the claims of fact and fault. But here I had an inside-out opportunity to explore the shifting, multisided experience of what was "true" without the limitations and opacities of legal testimony. As a writer, I wondered: If Ms. P were to sue him, would Dr. S's anger with himself—I assumed he was angry, as all doctors are experts in self-recrimination—get directed at her, or would it make him want to quit the profession? It wasn't just his anger that I was wondering about; it was hers too.

I assumed anger would be central to what I would hear from Ms. P. Aristotle described anger as "a desire accompanied by pain for an imagined retribution on account of an imagined slighting." Aristotle used the word "imagined" twice in his definition to emphasize that only the angry person's view matters; not the perpetrator's assessment, or the facts, which might not even be agreed on. But I was also curious to learn how Dr. S had responded to his patient's predictable fury or to his own self-criticism.

I was even more interested in how this surgeon and this patient might have negotiated the question of forgiveness, which I had come to think could be the great antidote for anger. Each might have agreed to speak to me to plead their case, to cast or dodge blame, but I hoped that these two had, at least for the time being, reached a kind of equilibrium. Speaking with them, I knew I would have to make sense of the fragility of the patient-doctor relationship, the evanescence of memory, and the literalness of the damaged body.

When I received their invitations to visit and talk, I was certain I would learn something important, something life-changing, if and when we spoke. I hoped I would. I needed to change my life.

Forgiveness

I was on my way to see the surgeon and the patient a week later, in a hurry to hear their stories. Although I was certain that similar medical mishaps were happening all over America, in the most tragic and final cases—when the patient died—one could learn only the doctor's version, and not privately, and only by reading the transcript of a court proceeding. It seemed a rare good fortune that I might hear from both parties in the aftermath of a (nonlethal) clinical accident. Each knew that I planned to speak with the other.

I planned to see P first. I was instinctively on her side. I was always willing to blame doctors. From the start of my career I had collected "bad doctor" stories, perhaps as a means of magical self-protection. If I collected enough of them, if I knew all the things that could go wrong, I would avoid mishap in my office with my patients, I'd imagined, but clearly this shield had recently failed me.

Maybe I was just another Dr. S; not as bad, not a disfigurer, but newly mistake-prone. Maybe I imagined that meeting Dr. S would be a chance to cross-examine him. Maybe this was a way to cross-examine myself, a new protagonist in a bad doctor story. Was it the mistake that mattered, or how one made sense of it in the aftermath? I was drawn to meet them for reasons I couldn't completely explain at the time. They lived three hours north, in Salem, home of the witch hunt.

I arrived at 8 A. M. at her small Cape house on a subdivision street without curbs. The house had an unkempt, yellowed lawn, but at the end of the slate front walk there were window boxes waiting for flowers. When I rang the doorbell, I heard a simple two-note chime inside the house. A tall, heavyset woman in her early fifties wearing a floral blouse opened the door and welcomed me in a high-pitched voice. She had big wild eyes that did not quite meet mine; she held her head almost sideways, obscuring the disfigured part of her face from me.

Ms. P was immediately chatty, asking about my drive, telling me how glad she was that I'd contacted her, letting me know her daughters might come over later. As I followed her into the house, she gave me looks over her left shoulder that were so thankful, so absurdly at odds with the reason for my visit, which she must have seen as an act of kindness, but to my mind was purely self-interest. I knew right there—amid the din of her talk—that the tenor of her thank-you said something about her that I would need to understand if I were to comprehend her reaction to her injury. I thought for a moment that this whole visit was ill-advised.

I followed her into a low-ceilinged living room crowded with overstuffed furniture that pressed its feet into tan wall-to-wall carpeting. Glass cabinets contained tiny teacups and crow-eyed porcelain dolls. I sat on the couch that looked out to an above-ground pool still covered in the middle of April and surrounded by a chain-link fence and, beyond it, a small rectangular plot separated from the neighbors by another chain-link fence. P handed me an old photograph album she'd put out on the table in front of the couch. "You'll see what I looked like before," she said, as she quickly went into the kitchen. It was as if she wanted my first serious consideration of her to be based on who she'd been before surgery. She came out with a cup of coffee for me (creamer and sugar bowl on the same silver tray) and a dish of Mallomars, a favorite cookie from when I was a boy and which I had forgotten existed. I was immediately returned to the kitchen of my childhood suburban house on a street much like this one, and I remembered the molded plastic tray of packaging the Mallomars sat in, how I was always surprised how much bigger than other cookies they were and how few there were, each in its own grooved inlay, apart from its neighbor. My father used to take the one I gave him and dunk it in coffee. It would drip on the way to his mouth.

Ms. P had brought herself nothing to drink. She stood over me, and her head lolled ever so slightly to the right, her chin tucked down as if she was shy. I kept trying to get a good look at her face, but she was a master at angling it away. Was my eagerness to stare into her face rude, unkind? Or was it a gesture of respect for pain she endured? It was easier to see the stains on her blouse below the right collar, suggesting she dribbled from one corner of her mouth. She was wearing rectangular black glasses on a chain and no makeup. I'd opened the album to a random page, trying to find her among the photos of family and friends. She left the room again, and when she came back she handed me a worn manila folder four inches thick and compressed by a rubber band. "I thought at some point you'd want to see my medical record," she said. I knew from our earliest email that she was a pediatric nurse and thus understood the value of any patient keeping copies of all medical documentation. I wondered if her being a medical provider herself, one who could make costly mistakes, had affected her behavior toward Dr. S. But still it surprised me to get handed these pages because it suggested to me that she wanted my medical opinion about what had befallen her, or that she was thinking about suing and knew that any attorney would ask for these records and just wanted me to understand how organized and prepared she was if she decided to proceed in that direction. It occurred to me that she saw me as a doctor, not as an ordinary visitor, and that was probably the reason she'd invited me to her home. In a way, this was another medical visit for her. She was used to dealing with doctors. She was also used to being a patient, I gathered from the thickness of the folder. But she wasn't my patient. I hadn't come to evaluate her medical care. I'd never considered that she was going to ask me to assess it so directly, if that's what she doing. I was planning to keep my opinions to myself.

When she finally sat down across from me,. I could see that half her face was caught in a twitch, lopsided. Her right cheek was slack, immobile; the right corner of her mouth drooped. Her left cheek trembled when she attempted to smile. I could see her considering me as I finally registered the damage.

It was hard to put myself in the place of this woman who woke up after surgery different from the way she'd gone to sleep.

"I used to check if the lump I'd first noticed two months before had grown. By the day of the surgery, I'd begun touching the skin just under my right ear several times an hour. Forefinger to earlobe had become a habit." P's nails were bitten down and she had a ring with a green stone on her middle finger. Her necklace dangled a gold wishbone.

"I'd always thought highly of Dr. S. Whenever we called in a consult to his office from the nursery, unlike every other plastic surgery office, his staff never asked what the patient's insurance was. He was one of only a few surgeons at our hospital willing to see patients without insurance. I've always been impressed by that. It meant a lot to me. He doesn't have the typical plastic surgery kind of office. It's regular, low key; it's not like those with gorgeous vases and beautiful paintings. There's no pretense in his; you'd never know it was where a plastic surgeon worked. He was my first and only choice to do the biopsy and, later, the surgery.

"At that first visit he mentioned that the lump might involve the parotid gland. A 'tumor'—that's what I remember him calling it—I immediately believed it was a cancer. That would be just my luck. Life was just starting back up five years after the divorce that ended my twenty-eight-year marriage."

She began to tell me the story she'd probably told many times before.

The pillows on her couch were as soft and rounded as the Mallomars. One framed needlepoint sampler on the wall said, "Laughter is the Best Medicine." The irony of this seemed cruel: it was probably very hard to laugh when your face was askew.

"At my gurney in the pre-op area on the day of the surgery, behind my blue curtain as I put on a johnnie, I remember thinking that the hospital's endless worry about compliance with the new federal HIPAA laws concerning health information privacy was hilarious; in this one big open room, you could hear everyone and everything. One patient was preparing for gastric bypass. Another, a nun, was having something done to her lung.

"A nurse I knew pulled open the curtain, asked how my Christmas had been two days before, and came in with a thermometer, pushing before her the machine to take my blood pressure. The nurse said she liked having Dr. S do the first case of the day at 8 A.M. because he was always on time. She asked if I had someone to pick me up when the operation was over.

"Dr. S entered the curtained area wearing scrubs, and chit-chatted for a few minutes. He told me, 'I'm going to get the tumor out.' He marked the surgical site just in front of my right ear with a black pen. He carried the surgical consent on a clipboard.

"'We should go over a few things,' he said. He let me hold the clipboard with the form. 'Do you want me to tell you about the bad things that could happen?' he asked me.

"'No, no, I trust you,' I remember answering."

Before she began the story of her "tumor" and surgery, she'd told me about her divorce, about her work in the nursery and how she was the staff member who offered to deliver the news to the parents of infants who died, and I'd realized that P thought of the world as a place that included physical decay, illness, death, and a limited control over fortune. She had a determination, and an ability to face difficult situations, that made me immediately think of her as a kind of optimist.

I drank two cups of coffee and finished four cookies. When I realized that she hadn't eaten or drunk a thing, presumably because of her embarrassment of eating or drinking in front of me (the stains on her blouse), I felt ashamed for enjoying my treat. I asked if I could take the folder of her medical record to review at home (she told me she had three copies) and come back to see her again soon, that I was due across town to see S. She was disappointed. She had set aside her entire day for me. She was eager to set another date.

As I was leaving, I reconsidered my initial impression. Did I have my first read of her exactly backward? Was her willingness to tell her surgical tale merely a sad consolation? Was her tone not optimistic but, rather, one of resigned acceptance in light of the futility to protest the loss of function of half of her face? Perhaps what I was hearing was the residue of reconciliation that included both optimism and consolation. Still, she emanated a kind of metaphysical forgiveness. I wanted my patients to forgive me.

From time to time over the past thirty years, I have pulled the copy of my father's death certificate from my desk drawer and looked at it. Each time, I felt an urge to smash something. But at the same time I felt so weak I could barely lift my arms. I would put my hands on the desk and lay my forehead on them and imagine driving to the office of this doctor who had signed the certificate, my father's longtime general practitioner, the man who "killed" him. I use the word "killed" as shorthand for my lifelong feeling that "not enough was done" when my father arrived in the emergency room with heart failure or, in my worst moments, that a mistake was made, that his doctor had been negligent. I had never forgiven him.

The doctor would have been an old man by time I would have found my way to him. Still, I imagined he would answer the door in slippers, as if I were an expected family member or visiting nurse. I would hide my hostility in order to get inside his house to explain my errand: to hear the events of my father's last night. He would be friendly, vulnerable, as if he was doing a good deed, although he was long past being a doctor. He wouldn't be agitated at all by my presence, as it would have been twenty years since he spoke of individual patients with anyone. He would remember my father, whom he had known for decades, and he would say how sorry he was that my father had died when I was so young, which was in no way an apology. He would not be protecting some long-held secret; he would simply not remember a thing about that last night.

On my drive across town to hear S's account, I thought about my low view of surgeons. In studies, the average length of time of a surgical office visit (preoperative, postoperative, routine follow-up) is about thirteen minutes, 25 percent briefer than an internist's. Taking a patient's history takes about three and a half of those minutes. The questions a surgeon uses are typically close-ended and answered yes or no—Have long have you had that? Does it hurt? A mechanic's diagnostic list. The physical examination takes about three minutes and is focused on body parts—the abdomen, the breasts; in P's case, the cheek. The education and counseling part of the average visit takes about five and a half minutes and is information-laden: the procedure is described, along with treatment alternatives (if the surgeon is being fully transparent), and the possible risks. There are usually some brief patient questions and some checking to see if the patient understands. The final minute of the thirteen is a review of next steps, plans, and the next appointment's timing. Less than 10 percent of a visit is devoted to lifestyle issues such as how the patient's work has been affected by the underlying problem or, postoperatively, by the surgery itself, and this line of conversation is more likely to be initiated by the patient; psychosocial issues (the patient's emotions or state of mind) constitute 1.3 percent of the average visit. Overall, surgeons talk about 50 percent more than their patients during the visit.

This workflow breakdown was different from my interactions with my primary care patients and was one of the reasons I had chosen not to become a surgeon. I had seen early on in my career that at least half the agony of a patient's condition was the inability to communicate his or her internal state; shorter visits made this nearly impossible. My role as a doctor was to act as an interlocutor and, by spending more time on a history, eventually make my way to a diagnosis. This is the work of an internist. Yet there were things I'd learned from studies of surgeons. Positive statements from the surgeon—approval, laughter, humor, support, encouragement—are ten times more common than statements of concern or worry; surgeons are optimistic and cheerful. Because I asked for more historical details, my longer visits were probably less positive and more upsetting experiences for some patients, despite my trying to evince concern and empathy. Surgeons are swift and efficient, and my low view of them was overgeneralized; one of my best friends was a sweet and caring eye surgeon whom I still ridiculed ("You must only have time to look in one of their eyes") for seeing sixty office patients a day when I managed fifteen.

In fact, for surgeons there is no correlation between the duration of a routine visit and malpractice claims history, as there is for primary care physicians. "Patients visiting surgeons may be seeking advice from a technical expert and may expect a businesslike manner," one communications expert speculates. So extensive communication with patients may not be important for surgeons, or not as important as I thought it should be. Except when things go wrong.

His three-story medical office building had narrow hallways, and doctors' names on bronze plaques on the wall to the left side of every thin door. His office was empty of patients at midday. The furnishings were plain, worn, the color scheme brown on brown. S came into the waiting area to shake my hand, a small pale man in his fifties with a hot palm, clear blue eyes, and soft, scuffed tan shoes. He had boyishly floppy brown hair with an out-of-style length, parted on the side. I followed him back toward his office. His secretary offered me tea, and as at P's house, I drank alone, across the pale wooden desk from a man who didn't have caffeine during the afternoon of a workday.

"When she came to have her biopsy stitches out, I told her that she had a benign histiocytoma, a very unusual noncancerous tumor. We talked about what her options were. Whether, because it was benign, we could leave it alone. Or whether, because it was growing and noticeable, we should do more. I told P the mass was a centimeter beneath the superficial lobe of the parotid gland—with the parotid there are two lobes, you may remember from your Anatomy class, the superficial and the deep, and in the middle is the facial nerve and all its branches—that it was bigger and deeper than I expected, so if we needed to take this out completely, we needed to do it under different conditions, in an operating room where I have better control, better lights, better instruments, and she's asleep.

"Her decision was to go ahead and remove it. She was very sure of what she wanted."

He had a soft voice and slow, careful movements. He was not the typical optimistic, cheerful surgeon. He spoke to me in a teacher's posture, seated but leaning forward. He was solemn, peaceful. Papers were strewn messily across his small desk and covering part of his phone: operative reports, announcements of committee meetings, letters from hospital administrators, a textbook. The office was only big enough for the desk, our two chairs, a bookshelf, and a small round table covered with more of the debris of a medical life—journals, half-written notes. He would never bring a patient into this office for a conversation. It was really a storage area.

I expected S to be cautious. He didn't know me. Even though I'd reached out to him through someone who did, I was a stranger arriving on a spring morning with an unknown agenda. I didn't understand why he would talk to me.

I liked that he had discussed options with P, uncertain of what to recommend. I could feel myself swinging over to his side; I saw doctor and patient in opposition in that moment, although neither had yet, in my short time with them, expressed antagonism toward the other.

In the short drive across town, I had felt myself eager to catch him admitting to a crime in some coded way. Maybe because I wanted to collect another bad doctor story. Maybe because I had a sheaf of medical records with his name and signature on them, sitting in the back seat of my car. That pile of papers made me feel like a detective. If he admitted to nothing, I would go through her medical records and find the evidence of his wrongdoing, I had already decided. As I was shuttling between patient and doctor, I wondered if he and P had discussed my intentions; I didn't really have a sense of the current state of their relations.

"P and I were friends before she became my patient. She took care of my kids in the nursery twenty years ago," S said after I told him I'd just been to see her. The Venetian blinds covering the window beside his desk were down.

"I think about any surgery before I do it. I think about where I'm going to make the incision. What I'm going to see. How I will do one or another part. I go through the entire procedure."

His was the voice of a man who'd had practice speaking about difficult topics. Was I this contained when I spoke with patients? I didn't think so. It was hard to reconcile my manner with his, although we shared one large and tricky requirement of being a doctor: we were the constant bearers of unfortunate news. Sitting across from S, I was every patient who was trying to understand what had gone amiss during a medical encounter. I was also every doctor who'd done his job and affected the lives of patients in ways he would never quite understand.

I'd come to hear his story (he'd set aside an hour before the afternoon's patients started to arrive), but I realized as he'd been talking that *I* wanted to confess. I wanted him to listen to a five-minute confession that would cure my guilt over my two patients. I wanted to be absolved by this solid, serious, careful doctor. S didn't need to know anything about me to bring about my cure. He only had to be sympathetic. It was the process—the listening itself—that would effect the cure, right? Isn't this what I always told my students? But this was laughable; any cure would be illusory.

"This is the part I remember vividly," he said. "The morning of surgery, it was a Thursday, two days after Christmas, I go in to see P pre-op at the SurgiCenter. She's very nervous about the operation, although she knows she should be able to go home by the afternoon. I ask her, 'Do you want me to go over all the bad things that happen during this operation?' She says no. I said okay, figuring since she was a nurse, she knew what was at stake here. And then we went into surgery, and the surgery was difficult. I remember it being difficult."

Was he also about to confess to me? Was this why he was talking to me? It didn't feel that way. S seemed too peaceful, too calm in his telling. I expected, I wanted, agitation.

But the rest of the hour with Dr. S was taken up by his recounting his training, his various roles at the hospital, and finally some of the details of P's case. He was interrupted twice by his secretary poking her head into the room to mention messages that had come in that morning. I didn't have time to ask him the deeper questions that had been weighing on me. But we agreed I could come back a week later.

—————

I read the surgical report the night that I returned from my first visits with S and P. It was near the end of the chart notes P had given me.

POSTOPERATIVE DIAGNOSIS:
    Spindle cell tumor of right neck
OPERATION: Excision of spindle cell tumor
    with superficial inferior parotidectomy
ANESTHESIA: General
INDICATIONS: Ms. P is a 54-year-old woman
    who presents with a diagnosis of spindle
    cell tumor. I suspect that this is in the
    parotid. Given the diagnosis, she has elected
    to proceed with complete excision.
PROCEDURE: The skin incision was made in the
    preauricular crease and carried down through the
    prior scar from the biopsy. A skin flap was then
    elevated anteriorly, including the SMAS. The
    mass was easily identified and seemed to be in
    the superficial lob of the inferior portion of the
    parotid. Therefore, dissection of this structure was
    taken out. We were able to get completely around

Forgiveness

the tumor with what seemed to be an appropriate border of normal tissue. Care was taken before dividing any tissues to test to make sure that this did not contain the facial nerve. Several times the nerve was isolated and avoided. The facial vein also remained intact on the inferior surface of this resection. After complete removal of the tumor, a drain was placed and exited out a separate stab wound. The wound was then closed in layers. This mass was closed with a Vicryl suture, and the skin was closed with 6-0 Prolene. Steri-strips were then applied. She was then awakened and taken to the recovery room in good condition.

There was no mention of a complication.

PART 2

I returned to Salem seven days later, the last week of April. I sat again on P's couch and this time she brought us each a glass of lemonade with a straw. I thought the straw, unwrapped and standing in the glass except for that last bit of paper on the top, was a way of handling the awkwardness of the disparity between my ease in drinking and her difficulty. I looked out the window at the pool and its blue tarpaulin cover. She sat across from me in a small gray chair that seemed undersized, as if it was a miniature pony carrying an adult.

She started in quickly again. She told me that she woke up in the main recovery room with a terrible headache. Her right cheek was numb, she presumed from the Novocain. She heard a doctor talking to a patient about a tumor in his belly and thought: that poor man. She was dizzy and wanted to clear her head in order to go home. She remembered looking at the clock, not having her glasses on, and seeing "11:00." She was supposed to have been home by noon. She didn't realize that she had double vision until a nurse told her it was actually 1 P.M. When the nurse said, "Give me a smile," she gave what she thought was a smile and fell back to sleep.

When she next woke, two nurses helped her into a chair in the recovery room. She felt horrible; she was shocked at how bad she felt, but she was set on going home. She just had to wait until the awful general anesthesia was metabolized. She was grateful she wasn't retching.

"I sat in a lounge chair, and the nurse asked, 'Would you like a drink?'" The nurse (who, P told me, is no longer working at the hospital, "which is a good thing") offered her a sip of ginger ale. "Of course, I'm thirsty, I had a tube down my throat. I tried to drink from a cup and the ginger ale rolled down one side of my face and onto the johnnie. I couldn't drink. I was thinking: Am I not with it enough to drink? I couldn't understand why my mouth wasn't coordinated. When would the Novocain wear off? Was that why I couldn't feel the right side of my face? Did it have something to do with the wicked headache that wouldn't stop?

"The nurse said, 'I'm going to get your kids, they've been frantic.' I didn't quite understand. They didn't have to be frantic,

I thought, I'm fine. I didn't realize they had been waiting over five hours to see me. The nurse disappeared into the family waiting area and brought in Kate and Lauren and the baby. When they came around the corner, my daughter burst into tears.

"The baby took his finger, put it to the right corner of my mouth, pulled it up, and screamed, 'Gommie,' his name for me. I'm thinking, Why did he do that? He was trying to help me smile. That's how I found out."

P paused and I set the cup of ginger ale on my knee in a moment of respect. P still had not taken a sip of hers.

"All these people I work with start to come by, and there is a look of horror on people's faces. What I found out later was what they all thought: that I'd stroked. The nurse was rubbing my Kate's back saying, 'Your mom is going to be okay.'"

"During the operation, I saw the nerve and was careful to protect it," S said to me when I arrived at his office that second afternoon. I'd told him that I had come from seeing P, who had described for me the moment she learned something had gone wrong during surgery. "I thought there could be some transitory damage, she would have a funny smile for a while, but that should go away. That would come from pulling and testing the nerve during surgery. It's called neuropraxia, some transient swelling, a short-term malfunction of the nerve from trauma, swelling, or inflammation. I figured that was the worst-case scenario."

It was hard to imagine myself as a surgeon who saw the evidence of his mistake and didn't know how it had happened. But it wasn't difficult to imagine how trying it was for him to recover from what he'd done.

"I get her to the recovery room. I do the paperwork until she's more awake. I look at her and ask her to smile, so I can see what's going on, and she has an obvious small defect. Her smile's crooked. That's the nerve I was worried about. Remember when Carol Burnett smiled funny for a while? She had a facelift and they hit that nerve."

I didn't remember Carol Burnett's smile, and I'd never really paid attention to her as a television personality—she was too loud and annoying—although I remembered my father and mother enjoying her.

"When you lift the skin up, tiny branches of the facial nerve are very superficial and she must have had one cut. I do facelifts. To avoid it, you have to be careful in the way you dissect. You know what to look for and where to look. You test everything before you cut it. When I see P's funny smile, I'm thinking, it's all right; she has a little neuropraxia, I knew it might happen. I wish it hadn't happened, and my heart sunk a little bit when it did. I tell her right there, and then I go out and tell her family."

Nearly half the public reports that they have experienced an error in a hospital in their own care or that of a family member; this figure excludes office settings where most of health care now occurs. Half of these reported inpatient errors had serious consequences: death, disability, severe pain. The seminal 2000 report from the Institute of Medicine *To Err Is Human* concluded that each year more Americans die as a result of medical errors made in hospitals than as a result of injuries from automobile accidents. Among possible causes of medical errors, the public considers the three most important causes (1) health professionals not having enough time with patients, (2) health professionals overworked, stressed, or fatigued, and (3) failure of health professionals to work together or communicate as a team.

Doctors overestimate the chance of being sued when they make a mistake. They believe 60 percent of negligent adverse events lead to lawsuits. This is thirty times higher than the actual risk. Malpractice claims represent, according to authors of a review of the subject, "a unique convergence of circumstances that invariably include communication, documentation, and interpersonal issues."

Still, each year, one out of every thirteen American doctors is involved in a malpractice claim. Dr. S performs plastic surgery, which is a high-risk specialty; one in seven plastic surgeons is currently facing a lawsuit. By the age of forty-five, 88 percent of high-risk specialists face their first claim; by the age of sixty-five, that number rises to an estimated 99 percent. Only one in four claims leads to a settlement or a trial resolution, but that generates more than ten thousand malpractice payments each year.

At the time of Ms. P's surgery, Dr. S had never been sued.

My father died of heart failure in an emergency room in the middle of the night when I was thirteen years old. His primary care doctor had come in to meet him when called. The medications used to treat heart failure today are surprisingly similar to those used the night my father arrived forty-five years ago: diuretics, nitrates. His initial vital signs in the emergency department were not awful according to his medical record from that night, which I keep in my desk drawer; he deteriorated under their watch. Did his doctor underestimate the initial symptoms? Did he miss a precipitating cause? Did he not act aggressively enough?

I had always blamed my father's doctor for malpractice. His was the first entry in my bad doctor story collection. More than four decades later I was still furious with and resentful of him, this man who had been with my father the night he died, a man whom I'd once met and who himself had long since died. I was also terrified of becoming like him, a doctor who made mistakes and lost patients without facing the truth. I was angry at a ghost; I was still working out or over the past. I had gone to Salem to examine anger and forgiveness.

I was my father's representative, a wronged third party, a son, a doctor, blamed and blaming. I had seen P twice and I was still waiting for her to tell me she hated Dr. S.

As I studied the dry leaves tumbling over the pool's blue cover, P said, "My upset started, I think, with hearing the nurse in the recovery room say to someone on the phone, 'She feels like she can't go home.' That nurse could have stopped the discharge process herself rather than putting it on me. *She* doesn't think she can go home? How about *I* don't think she should go home.

That nurse should have called the doctor when she saw my face wasn't right and said, 'She needs to be admitted.'"

I was surprised that she was so unhappy with her nursing colleague, but I realized that the nurse was the first person she saw upon waking and was therefore the initial target.

"Before I leave the recovery room, I need to know what I look like. I ask a nurse who's a good friend to bring me a mirror. I looked and it was horrible. I remember thinking it was a bad dream. My right eyelid was not shutting. I was totally shifted. My nose went to one side.

"I thought I was going to pass out. My friend was holding on to me, crying. I looked in the mirror and thought, who am I? I said out loud, 'What the hell happened?'

"I don't remember even seeing Dr. S in recovery. He said later that he told me my face was a little shifted. I asked him what I did when he told me, and he said I just shook my head. If I really got it, I would have burst into tears, which means I didn't really understand what had happened until my grandson came in.

"I do think Dr. S learned a bitter lesson. He learned that if your patient isn't with it, you'd better wait to tell them news. Don't leave too soon, because the patient will feel abandoned. He should have said to the nurse, 'When she's more awake, call me back.' But he needed to get out of that recovery room right then, I'm sure."

"I go over the whole operation again in my head as soon as I leave the recovery room," S said. "There's a famous paper written by a plastic surgeon about how to do a safe parotidectomy in a half hour. I read it when I was a resident. I remember it not only because he was proposing a preposterous length of time, but also because the author goes over all the maneuvers you do to protect the facial nerve. You identify it. You follow it along and never lose sight of it. You test before you cut. All the things that anyone who does this surgery knows how to do. In a normal patient you can see the full length of the nerve, but in P's case it went in and out of the tumor. Yes, part of it traveled behind the tumor, and until I took it out I couldn't see it. Is it possible that I cut it? It's possible. I didn't think so at the time and I still don't think so."

Although I was always willing to blame doctors, as I listened to S's surgical preparation and his description of the operation, I began to doubt that he had made an egregious surgical error.

"I didn't know how long the operation had gone until I'd come out of surgery and saw the clock. I had people waiting for me in my office across the street. I like to be on time.

"But as I went toward my office I started thinking, What did I do wrong? I didn't do anything wrong. I do the operation in my head over and over and over again. At that point I was still confident in how I did the procedure. I knew I took my time and was careful. I did it the way I should have. All the while I have this hope that what happened will only be an inconvenience for P. I'd obviously never seen this before in one of my patients."

I imagined him returning to this office that day after his operative morning, greeting his staff, telling them he'd be out to see his first afternoon patient in a few minutes ("Please apologize to them that I'm running late"), maybe taking a few bites of a cheese and tomato sandwich he'd brought from home, sealed in clear wrap, sitting at this very desk where we were speaking almost three years later. Would his secretary have had a sense from his scrubbed and full face and his tardiness that something had gone wrong in the OR? He wouldn't have dwelled on it that afternoon with a lineup of patients waiting to be seen and taken care of.

S described each day as a series of rituals. He had a regularity and a way of doing things from the time of his first morning coffee to the order in which he packed his briefcase to go home. He no longer remembered why or when he formed these habits, but the present had always looked like the past. Now he needed to free himself from the effects of the past. He had learned two related lessons: *The next time is not necessarily like the time before*, and *What you thought you'd learned doesn't always apply*.

"Here I am, I'm the one," S said to me this last week in April. "Nobody else did anything to her." He had tears in his eyes. "I can't explain how it happened. Did I do something wrong? I went to her hospital room late that afternoon on the day of the surgery; we were alone; her daughters weren't there. I told her exactly what I saw during the operation and what I was seeing that day. The one thing we had was that we were friends and I felt I could tell P what I was seeing, and that I didn't know why it was happening. I wasn't afraid to say that I didn't understand what was going on, as you might be afraid to admit to most patients. I told her I would take care of her and we'd do what she needed." He started to cry. He used the back of his hand to wipe away the tears.

I was waiting for S to say something more than "Did I do something wrong?" I was waiting for him to admit he'd made a mistake.

To excuse a person is to hold him not responsible, even while his action is recognized as wrong. To excuse a person is to judge that he acted involuntarily. Excusing means the injured party is not taking the injuring act as a sign of any inherent viciousness.

By contrast, to forgive a person is to assume that he is responsible for the wrongdoing; to forgive suggests that the wrong was done in some sense voluntarily. This voluntariness creates a different moral relation between wrongdoer and the wronged than involuntariness does.

S had no bad intent. He did not set out to injure P; he did not know there was a problem during the operation. It was an unexpected complication. The wrongdoing was involuntary. So does the moral relationship between an injured patient and her doctor call out for forgiveness, based on S's responsibility, or for excusing, as P's facial paralysis was certainly unintended?

Negligence (a medical malpractice term) suggests voluntariness. S had, after all, suggested this operation (although P had insisted on "taking it out" originally); he had performed the surgery in a certain way; the surgery had gone on longer than planned. But of course, the outcome was unintended; he hadn't harmed P on purpose; the wrongdoing was not intentional. The change in their relationship when P woke up arose in part because of the complexity of this concept of voluntary (versus involuntary) action.

Still, it would be hard for her not to be angry. It would be hard *not* to hold him responsible, even if he had not acted out of negligence. That was the predicament.

I wondered how many months it would be before the pool tarp came off and P could start swimming outside. P still hadn't sipped her ginger ale, and I was self-conscious about sipping mine.

"I spend a night in the hospital and the next morning, breakfast comes and there's coffee, and I'm a big coffee drinker," P told me. "The nurse takes the coffee cup away and says, 'You can't drink this.' I said, 'I have to have coffee.'

"I asked her to give me a straw and I stuck it in. My dad had Parkinson's and he always drank with straws. My sisters say, 'At least you don't rinse them out like he did.' My father would keep a straw for the day.

"Dr. S came in before eight. He sat on the edge of the bed. My speech was bad; I didn't know how to talk anymore, but it was the headache from the anesthesia that bothered me most. I ate some oatmeal and it was dribbling out but I got some down.

"I don't know how Dr. S walked into that room up on the surgical ward that morning. There was a lineup in my room already at that hour. My two kids, coworkers, friends. He sat next to me. He spoke only to me, but other people were listening. He said everything went fine during surgery. He said there was a lot of bleeding. I can't remember if he said that it was bigger than he expected or it was harder to get out or both. He said it really wanted to stay in there."

P gave me an eye roll and resettled on her miniature gray chair.

"It was Friday morning and I wanted to go home but he wanted me to stay a while longer. We didn't have a long discussion. There were too many ears in the room. If a physician needs to talk to a patient after that kind of event, then the setting has to be right." For the first time, I heard P's tone turn to a nurse's instructional tone, rather than a patient's voice.

"It would have been worse if he'd come in and said, 'You all have to leave,' but for a physician to walk into a room full of people isn't an easy thing either. You could feel everyone wanting to talk, but no one would. He said he'd see me later in the day, and I told him again I was ready to leave. Mind you, I'm not even eating yet. He said, 'You're gonna be okay.' He kept saying that.

"I asked him later, Why did he keep telling me that? And he said, 'Because I needed you to be.'"

"Nobody goes into this profession wanting to hurt people. That's the last thing that we want," S said as he stood and straightened his white coat and readied himself for the lineup of waiting patients.

"Once in a lifetime. It's the only time this has ever happened in all the facial surgeries I've done. All during my office hours that first day, I was an optimist hoping P's problem would go away. I'm worrying about her, I'm starting to feel bad, but I think it's going to be a minor inconvenience for a couple of months.

"I'm also thinking this is a disaster. How could I have possibly done this?

"Friday evening, after I finish in the office, I went over to see her again. She's in a room, in pretty good spirits, not in any pain. Her daughters are there and I can tell that they are pissed, giving me the evil eye. But they don't say anything. They are clearly upset. This is almost thirty-six hours after surgery and P still has asymmetry; you can see it when she speaks. We talked about it again: this is a nerve I saw during the operation, I tested for it to see that it worked, I'm sure I avoided it, this is a temporary thing, and I expect that your function will come back in months.

"I go home. I feel terrible. I don't know what to do; there's nothing I can do. I have a terrible night. For the second straight day, I didn't tell my wife, maybe because I was trying to pretend it didn't happen. Or if I don't say it out loud, I don't have to face it. Or maybe it was just hopefulness that things would get better."

"When he leaves on Friday night, there's anger in the room," P said as she cleared my lemonade and her own. "Both my kids say, 'We should get a lawyer. Something's wrong.' My oldest daughter, Kate, had already talked to her friend's husband who's a malpractice attorney. I looked at them and said, 'I just want to get better. No lawyer talk.' And off they went for the night. Angry."

Physicians, professional organizations' codes of conduct, ethicists, and the public seem to agree that physicians are obligated to disclose medical errors. The elements of the ideal disclosure are generally accepted to be (1) notification of an error, (2) a description of what happened, (3) a sincere apology, (4) acceptance of responsibility, (5) a description of steps to be taken to mitigate harm and correct the situation, and (6) assurance of an investigation to prevent recurrence.

Participants in a well-known study of medical errors were shown videotapes of physician-patient dialogues in three "mistake" scenarios: (1) after a delay in noticing a mammogram abnormality, (2) following a chemotherapy overdose of ten times the intended amount, and (3) after a slow response to pages for a patient eventually rushed to surgery. In each scenario, the researchers varied the apology type—full (personal and specific), nonspecific (I'm sorry your family member is so ill), and nonapology—and whether or not the physician accepted responsibility. A full apology and acceptance of responsibility were associated with better viewer ratings of the physician's handling of the incident, trust, and desire to have that physician as their own. But neither the type of apology nor the acceptance of responsibility was associated with the viewer's likelihood to sue.

Anger is swift and brief, and as a response to pain sometimes helpful, making the pain disappear for a moment. Other times anger cannot be overcome; Beatriz never returned to see me. My words in front of Dahlia were irrecoverable, unreachable, an error that led to an immutable result. It was too early to know whether I might still be exonerated by my other patients for my smaller, more recent errors.

Anger acutely distracts us from hurt and harm, but I imagined that whenever P looked into the mirror anger reared, as it would have for me if I'd been injured. I imagined her thinking as I would: My situation is stunningly unfair—what did I do to deserve this? If it had been me, this diminishment of capacities and prospects would have felt like a punishment. Even if S's action was unintentional, the result was unfair. She could take an "objective" view but still be angry. She had no part in bringing this deformity on herself.

Anger that continues, that is continually provoked over a long period, becomes resentment. Resentment is a second stage of anger, an afterburn. Resentment can be directed at a person or what he or she did. But the doctor *is* the action; to an individual patient, they are what they did. One can feel resentment even while not believing that the target of our resentment is really to blame.

Resentment also offers some satisfactions. It generates sympathy. There is the pride of forbearance and survival. Resentment presents the injured as standing shiningly in the right. The resentful person creates a narrative about the injury, the injurer, and the injured who becomes the victim, the wronged—such a narrative has a moral. At times, however, unchecked resentment consumes everyone, including its possessor.

Yet P had described her daughters, not herself, as angry. They, I knew, hated Dr. S and considered him "blameworthy." They had been after their mother to file a lawsuit from the first postsurgical hour. But had P ever been furious at S? I'd not heard anger or resentment in her voice; she had, seemingly, excused him? Whether she had forgiven him or not, did she believe he deserved punishment?

When I thought about P and about my father, I thought about the magnitude of the injury: Is death forgivable? And I felt bad that I was thinking of P's injury as minor, or less significant than what my father's doctor had done to him. And at the same time I began to feel that my two mistakes with patients, minor and reversible and impermanent, were therefore pardonable, at my least by myself.

PART 3

Most faces are defined by simple shapes and symmetry. Oval eyes, circular nostrils, the straight line of pursed lips. P's face was more complex. Since the surgery it had remained unbalanced, irregular, misshapen. If I hadn't spent six hours with her, I might have thought her cheek's twist made her look evil, the classic signs of untrustworthiness or menace. There was no geometrical simplicity to her face even three years later. But her big, clear voice was not anguished. She had made a new life.

I arrived for my third visit during the first week of May. The slate front steps and trim black railing were almost familiar. I was still taking time out of work—it had been almost a month—though I had checked in with my office to see if either of the patients I had mishandled had called to schedule new appointments, that is, had forgiven me. They hadn't and this disappointed me.

"My daughter Kate took me home and she stayed all day because she didn't want to leave me alone. When I get home it hits me. First of all, there are more mirrors. Second, I had set my bed up before I'd left for surgery, and had new PJs because I thought when I got home I'd want to take a nap in comfortable clothes. I remember thinking when my daughter led me into my house: you are not the same person as when you left.

"She brought a camera into my room that morning. Paul, her lawyer friend, was ready to call me, she said again. She tried to take pictures of me. I said, 'Don't. What are you doing?' She says, 'Paul said that we need to start taking pictures.' I didn't let her. She says, 'He butchered you.' I defended Dr. S. I said, 'No, he didn't.' She says, 'Why are you defending him?'

"Morning TV is very dangerous. I don't know if you know the commercials of James Sokolove, the malpractice attorney? Constant commercials about whether you've been misdiagnosed or are suffering from a medical injury. He has a lot of commercials. If you're sitting home, freaking out or depressed or angry, you know where to call."

I realized that as I had been driving north on that beautiful cloudless day, I'd been noticing things that sagged: telephone lines against the blue sky, broken storefront awnings, weeping willows.

"I didn't want anyone to know. I didn't want anyone to say, 'What a hack,'" S said to me that May morning when I stopped by his office after seeing P for what would be my final visit. He was almost whispering, as if I shouldn't tell anyone. He was more emotional, vulnerable, than he'd been at my earlier visits. Maybe remembering and retelling his story had made him more open with me. "I was worried about my career. Who is going to send their patients to see me anymore if something like this can happen? They'll hear about the complication and think, Let's send our patients elsewhere. I have no precedent for this. I've had complications, of course. I've had patients with bleeding after surgery. But you go back and take care of it and that's the end of it. I was totally unprepared for this.

"It's like losing someone. Something terrible has happened and you go through the Kübler-Ross stages. After that second day, I got depressed. I had no one to talk to about it. But I didn't want to talk to anybody. I felt I should quit my job, that I couldn't do this anymore. I couldn't sleep. I lost interest in all my activities. It was a gradual downslope after that."

"I'm about ready to quit mine," I said. "I've had some patient problems recently."

He didn't pick up on this invitation to ask me more. He was a quiet man with good manners. Maybe he didn't want to be intrusive. Maybe he didn't quite register that I was in a bad way too. Maybe, sensing my tone of self-pity, he didn't have the energy hear me out. Maybe he thought that continuing his story might help me.

"I had no confidence, and I became hyperalert to making any sort of mistake," S said in his soft voice. "Not being a confident surgeon is a bad state. You start second-guessing even the simplest things. I didn't cancel surgeries, but I was anxious about what would happen in each.

"Before, I was confident. I had good results. Patients were happy. That cycle was over. I thought I was never going to feel that again. From that day forward, I stopped doing parotid surgery. I didn't want to have this ever to happen to me or a patient again. I did my best and look what happened. So I'm obviously not fit to do this.

"I didn't stop facelifts, which have the same risk, which doesn't make sense, I know. It was an emotional decision. I tried to get through the day. That was all."

To begin the work of forgiveness, the offender must take six steps in the ideal case. I tried to assess how well S had accomplished these. First, S admitted to responsibility; if he had disavowed the act, then the truth could never be reached. Second, he repudiated the deed and promised to try to do better. Third, it was clear that he experienced and expressed regret at having caused the injury; his apology was a sign of respect for P. Fourth, he had committed to becoming the sort of person who will not inflict such an injury again, commitment through deed as well as words. Dr. S had decided never to do parotid surgery again, to leave this kind of surgery to other surgeons. These four steps constituted contrition. Fifth, in an exercise of sympathy, he had shown that he understood the damage done from P's perspective. He had heard P's account many times over these years, I presumed, each time with compassion. I could imagine him listening to her the first time, anguished, awaiting her outrage. Finally, S offered a narrative accounting for how he had injured her, and how that wrongdoing did not express the totality of his person. This account was not excuse-making, but a description of context.

These six steps S seemed to have taken were not part of a conscious therapeutic program he assigned himself; they happened naturally. And in response, these conditions might have been what allowed P, a victim, to see her offender more broadly, as someone more than an injurer.

I had reached out to those I had injured, to Beatriz and the others, but no one returned my calls. I wasn't going to run into them around town, as was the situation for Dr. S and Ms. P.

"I remember thinking, Why are we talking legal when we don't even know what happened to me?" P said that May morning of my third visit. "I said to my daughter, 'I'm gonna get better and I don't want to focus on what's wrong. I want to get better.' I think maybe because I work in Neonatal, I know that things go wrong and it's no one's fault. But society says, *When things go bad, someone is responsible.* Two of my siblings think, Life screwed us; the world owes us because things sucked in life. But I don't live my life like that. I've always been more compassionate. I felt the physician I chose for my surgery was not a nutcase (I've known some of those). He wasn't an unsafe practitioner.

"It continues to pit my daughters against me. They've never dropped the subject of lawyers."

I identified with her children, third parties who sought reparation from a doctor for a parent. If P had not survived, everything would have been different, I believed. They would have known nothing of Dr. S's thoughts or reactions, or his relationship with their mother, and they would have sued him.

I knew certain patients, and certainly one child, who considered my mistakes unforgivable.

"For the first three weeks I couldn't drive, I was so tired," P said. "Not only was I frustrated, I was shocked. I drove two hours to see a facial nerve specialist. On my way to her office the first time, I thought she could fix me. I thought she'd go back into my cheek and fix it."

When she tried to grin, her smile seemed to have jammed. But I could hear in her high, cooing voice that P was still hopeful.

"When Dr. H came in, I saw she was a kid, bouncy. She had already spoken with Dr. S extensively about the surgery. She said, 'You know this is a surgeon's nightmare.' Kate, who was with me that day, said, 'Well what about my mother?' Dr. H understood that it was my nightmare too, but that I had good potential. She sent me to bootcamp with her facial nerve physical therapist. A speech therapist started coming to the house three times a week. I cried every time he came.

"The therapist was teaching me how to form my words again, how to make my mouth move, because at that point I had no movement of my right upper lip. I was strictly talking from the left side of my mouth. You need your whole mouth to form words, and I was missing half. His exercises were like dog tricks.

Forming circles with my mouth, blowing a candle, holding the blow. Putting a finger inside my lip and making a circle. Trying to stretch the lip, pull the upper right lip to the right, trying to show teeth, massaging the lip with forefinger in and thumb on the outside. The big event was trying to eat. I had a whole routine I did three or four times a day. I practiced eating all day, little bits, soft foods, with my towel nearby for my drooling.

"I was starting to look better as my mouth did some wiggling. The sign that I was better was getting a pedicure. That was my first trip out alone about four weeks after surgery."

She had never exploded or raged at Dr. S she told me. Her calm contrasted so starkly with the difficulties of her life. She had been required to pull off some impossible feat in working out her feelings.

At thirteen, I had been vaulted into adulthood by my father's death and had not recovered in some ways. Thinking back on my medical career, I was preternaturally careful in all dealings with patients, afraid of accidents and mistakes, distressed by their slightest discontent. I wanted to be loved by patients. Yet over the years I had remained a boy in all my retellings of my father's last night, enraged as only a teenager can be as a defense against the emptiness. But in the month before I first drove to Salem, I had slipped across some sentimental divide; now I was the doctor who made the mistakes and I had gone looking for new defenses against all my strong feelings of upset. The doubleness of my Salem visits, going back and forth between P's optimism and S's melancholy, between my juvenile grief and my recent medical flaws and self-pity, left me confused about how I wanted to be seen, what disclaimers I wanted to post for the next patient I would care for.

***

"When P goes back to work after about a month, everyone says to her, 'Oh my God, what happened?'" S told me that May morning. "A week later, I get stopped by the chief medical officer of the hospital. He's an administrator, but still a practicing doc and he says, 'What the hell did you do to P?' I'm taken aback. I already feel terrible. I say, 'Listen, this is what I did. I've been over it a million times.' We have this conversation in the hallway. He's never said another word to me."

***

"Did I know the day that I got hurt that I would be permanently disabled? Did I know that my face would always be pulled over to one side? Although I was still weak, I went back to work after six weeks. I got no negative comments from staff, but I did overhear a patient tell another nurse, 'Mine is the one who looks like she had a stroke.' I usually addressed it with my patients early on; I'd tell them it looks like I'm a little twisted, but my brain is fine."

***

"I'm good at surgery. Except that time. It doesn't matter that I don't understand what happened," S said, accepting mystery, understanding the futility of looking for answers.

"I avoided my colleagues and they avoided me. I had leprosy. My friends at work wouldn't look me in the eye. They wouldn't have normal conversations with me. I got the feeling that they thought I was contagious, that it would rub off. Or they didn't know what to say to me. Or they didn't want to hurt my feelings. I didn't know what they were thinking."

He had become a bad doctor story, I thought.

"I became an untouchable. I didn't want to talk about it. I didn't want to relive it. I kept thinking I should quit, that I shouldn't see patients anymore. It sounds stupid, but I didn't know how to start seeking help. I thought it would be like falling off a horse. Just get back up and ride. Suck it up. Be a man. The attitude from surgical training. The surgical ABCs are Assess, Blame, and Criticize, and then move on.

"But I felt more and more isolated. Talk about being alone: I was a guy on a desert island at this point. No one to talk to. Feeling miserable. Seeing no way out. It was awful."

S was the one I'd come to blame, but everyone in his medical world already blamed him despite the six advances toward forgiveness he'd managed. Two years later he was still forlorn. I watched him shrink in his chair each time I asked him to speak about all this. Yet in the moral universe, he felt innocent to me.

"I felt alone. Except for Dr. S. He's never run on me," P said as I handed her back her medical file. "I've said to people, I didn't want to be adversarial. I was going to see him in the hallway. What was I going to do, run the other way? Or not talk? In the hall we'd both check to see if people were looking at us, asking each other what we were doing talking together."

I understood that both she and S were ashamed. And when they shared this shame, they had a solidarity.

"I told him I wanted to go to the hospital administration with suggestions and goals for how to take care of surgical patients. I thought, 'If I tell them what happened to me and how we could make the process better, we'd get it all fixed.' I wanted to tell them that sometimes the operating room extends beyond its walls. But the hospital said I needed representation if I wanted to speak with them, which thrilled my kids."

The work of forgiveness is bilateral. Just as seeking forgiveness required a series of steps from S, granting it required steps from P who had to get past her sense of having had something stolen to achieve true or ideal forgiveness. First, any resentment by P would have to be moderated or given up. Second, P, the injured party, had to enter imaginatively, sympathetically, into the role of offender and, through this reframing, revise her judgment of S. There is an ancient Greek word, *sungnome*, that means "to understand, to sympathize, to forgive"; it is a word that refuses to distinguish between thinking and feeling and captured what I'd heard from P. The third condition required that P drop any assumption of moral superiority over S. Fourth, P had to address S directly and grant forgiveness. It seemed, amazingly, as if she had performed all of these within days to weeks of the surgery. Was she morally obligated to forgive when S had taken the appropriate steps, or is forgiveness a gift?

The final step was that the injured should forswear revenge.

"My daughter's lawyer friend came to see me. He said, 'I've never met anyone like you. Most come to me because they're very angry and out for blood.' I told him I was not going to sue S. He said, 'In my line of work you never say you're *not* going to sue.'

"P wanted to meet with the hospital and me. She had a lawyer who was looking for some compensation to help with her post-op medical bills, the physical therapy, the eye doctor, hoping the hospital would kick something in. The hospital refused to meet with her without having their lawyers there. And they wouldn't have me there either, which P requested and I had agreed to. They assumed that when I was sued my insurance would take care of it. So they tried to put it all on me. They stonewalled and refused to meet with her because they didn't want to get in the middle of it. Until they were sued, they wouldn't offer to pay a thing."

"I told the hospital, I don't want to sue you. My goal was only that no one ever go through something this again. My lawyer met with Dr. S for twenty minutes in his office. She says she had never met a physician who would meet her without legal counsel. She recommended counsel but he said he didn't want one. She told him she had an expert opinion saying he did not do the surgery the right way. I don't know what he said to that. She came back and told me, 'He doesn't feel he did anything wrong.' I told her I wasn't surprised. No physician will stand there and say, 'I did it wrong.' But I wasn't looking for that. She genuinely believed he felt terrible this happened and he would do what it takes to make things better."

"After meeting P's lawyer, did I think I would be sued? Honestly, no." S offered a half-smile and reached over to pull the cord that lifted his Venetian blinds, showing us the gray May weather; it was still light out, the days were getting longer. "Because P came out and told me she wouldn't. If I was sued, so what? I was still going to care for her. She was my friend and it happened because of me. I wanted to see her through her recovery. I never got a lawyer, and if I had and they'd warned me to act differently with P, I wouldn't have listened. She knew what I was going through and I knew what she was going through because we talked.

"We'd always been honest with one another. When I was a new father and my babies were sick when they were newborns, she told me what was going on. How else can patients trust you if you're not honest with them? How else can you do this kind of work unless you're truthful?"

In my last hour with P she grew agitated and raised her voice for the first and only time during my three visits. "I never had a meeting with the administration. I never heard anyone from the hospital say to me, 'Take whatever time you need to get better. We're here for you and will do everything in our power for you.'

"No one said, 'Here's our best neurologist, here's our best speech and swallow therapist, here's the eye doctor—we'll make them available to you whenever you need.' I had to ask.

"I wrote them a letter offering solutions: an OR liaison person to address the family during surgery; another person who provides closer follow-up if an unexpected problem arises. I suggested that we use my medical record to educate staff. In my post-op note, Dr. S never mentions the asymmetrical smile. I leave the OR in mighty fine shape. I recommended that we train the recovery room nurses to ask patients what they remember after the doctor's left.

"The administrators at my hospital wrote back, 'We have to change things.' But the wheel turns very slowly."

"My preoperative risk discussion has changed," S said. "I take fewer things for granted. When I do surgery on another health care worker, I go through every risk as if they know nothing. I'll say, 'I know you may know more about this than other people, and I may be boring you, but these are the things I need to say out loud.' I'm more emphatic about telling them, and I say, 'Humor me. Listen.'

"When I hear about things in the hospital that go wrong, I offer to talk with those doctors. If you're that doctor, right at the beginning you're not going to go out and say 'I need someone to share this with.' Someone has to come to you. I go up to them, and most of the time they know my story, I tell them I understand the feelings they're having and if they want to talk, I'm here. We don't have to talk specifics, but how to get through it. Some take me up and some don't and deal with it themselves."

I had arrived in Salem believing there is a human need to turn sorrow unequivocally, insistently, ruthlessly to blame. My father's doctor had done nothing to me, but he'd done everything to me. My father's doctor would never apologize to me. He was long gone. My anger at him had been lodged deep inside me.

P never converted grief to rage. It had never occurred to her to do that; she knew S too well. Maybe, following his steps of guilt, regret, and remorse, P confirmed what she knew of S's character and believed that it warranted forgiveness. She knew he had done his best.

I was touched by her humor and honesty. She was not hard-hearted. Salvaging her dignity, she saw forgiveness as part of moral and spiritual growth.

As a writer, I had wanted to know what had happened between this surgeon and his disfigured patient, the chronology of events, and how life had changed for each in the aftermath, but now I wondered: Who is the object and who is the subject of a story about a medical error? S was benevolent, and in return he had been fortunate enough to make a mistake on someone who was naturally good and unafraid. She saw fellow humans as mirrors. If love and optimism are in you, you see it in others.

Forgiveness takes long effort. It is painful and contradictory and maddening. If he had survived, debilitated, would my father have rendered forgiveness, assuming his doctor apologized and met all the other conditions of pardon? Talking to P, I understood that I knew very little about my father who died when I was just a boy. But after these trips to Salem and weeks thinking about him, I had decided my father's character had been one of reconciliation and that should be enough for me. Perhaps forty-five years later it was time to absolve that doctor on my father's behalf, even if I couldn't immediately establish a steady state, even if on some days I would feel forgiveness and other days not.

I wanted Beatriz and the others to absolve me, and although they hadn't, I better understood the conditions necessary, and I was newly hopeful, which was enough to allow me to return to work.

"Whenever I see her, it hurts me. Every single time," S said as he walked me to his office door the final time. "She may not look bad any longer, but she won't eat in front of me. She has to use a straw. She has to have pureed food. She has to get Botox every ten weeks or her face is very pulled over. She still chokes from time to time. This is all my fault. And she's forgiven me, I know she has. But I haven't forgiven me. I know she cries a lot, although she tries not to do it when we talk. I try to be strong for her and I think she tries to be strong for me. I try not to cry in front of her either."

10

Kindness Matters

We all want to believe that a doctor's kindness matters for patient outcomes; *I* do. I'm convinced that when doctors are kind, patients do better. Now that I am back at work—Beatriz some years behind me, and still checking in with Dr. S and Ms. P—I want to tell you about four clinical studies that provide evidence for the effects of kindness and why it matters.

The first study involves homeless men and women. The homeless often lack primary care providers and commonly seek emergency room care. In an effort to slow the flow of costly return visits by the homeless, the administrators of one emergency department (ED) asked a research team to try something new in the delivery of care to this group. The researchers had trained college student volunteers to provide "compassionate contact" when a homeless person arrived for treatment at the ED. This involved nothing more than asking the volunteers to approach patients when they were waiting to be seen, to explain they were students thinking of careers in medicine, and then to have ordinary, nonmedical conversations, to share common experiences such as favorite television shows or family problems, and to listen attentively. That is, to be kind.

The doctors, nurses, and staff were told only that the hospital was now providing volunteers who would be available to speak with homeless patients as they waited for tests or received treatment during the long emergency room visits. The researchers then randomly assigned half of the arriving homeless patients to speak with a student volunteer; the other half would not get this extra company; all patients received the usual clinical care for their back pain, skin rashes, headaches. Over a four-month period, whenever homeless study participants assigned to the "compassionate contact" group returned to the ED, they saw a volunteer again; at each visit they answered questionnaires about the quality of care they received.

The researchers predicted two possible outcomes. First, that the extra contact would be so personally meaningful that homeless patients, seeking out these conversations, would *increase* their visits to the emergency room, not a result that the ED staff would like. Or, second, it was possible that kindness would lessen the number of visits because patient satisfaction improved, the homeless patients felt that their medical problems were solved, and they saw no reason to return for second and third evaluations and opinions.

The researchers found that repeat visits were 33 percent lower over the next year (at baseline, this population came in about once every other month) in the compassionate contact group compared to those who received usual care. Further, the homeless patients reported greater feelings of respect and courtesy, less frustration from any waiting times, and improved quality of care. Indeed, ED visits decreased as satisfaction increased. How can we explain these results? Perhaps the students, by demonstrating kindness through normal conversations, had promoted trust in the medical system, in the treatment given and the medical providers' opinions, that might suggest that no further treatment or return visits were needed. That is, the inclusion of a nonmedical interaction may have reinforced any reassurance given by doctors and nurses during regular care. I suspect the result was also due to a simpler element: the extra time spent and the informality of the conversation—a chat, a human exchange— produced a comforting effect. These two aspects of care—time and talk—these kindnesses, are at odds with the traditions and work pressures of rushed doctors, and this finding suggests what the medical encounter might include to have its best effect.

There could be a payoff if this simple decency were applied across a health system: happier patients; monetary savings if the homeless were uninsured and the ED received no payment for services rendered to them; fewer unnecessary return visits, freeing up staff time for true emergencies.

The researchers of this ED did not study whether their kindness intervention had any effect on *patient outcomes*. The hardnosed and unsentimental person might accept that kindness can improve the immediate postvisit satisfaction of homeless people, which might affect their future behavior and repeat visits, but could reasonably ask, Does kindness affect whether a patient judges her *health* as better?

A second study offers an answer. Following a serious accident that requires hospitalization and surgery, only about half of people get back to their prior type or level of work. Only a small percentage of these patients have recovered completely a year after hospitalization for severe trauma; even a year later most patients report significant functional impairment or mental health symptoms. In the shadow of these long-lasting problems, how patients perceive the effects of their often-extended hospital care on their long-term outcomes is important. In a study of hundreds of patients admitted to a trauma center after an injury, patients' ratings of their physician's empathy were associated with their perception of the treatment effectiveness, treatment satisfaction, and the treatment's effect on quality of life. Patients who found their surgeons more empathetic were functioning better, physically and mentally, a year after hospital release, a remarkable result.

One might think that the length of the hospital stay, or the number of surgeries—returns to the operating room are common—or injury severity might dominate patients' experience of their medical care. Yet the study suggested that better long-term patient outcomes after trauma surgery was in good part driven by better emotional care; the relational aspects of doctors and patients were determinative even in this high-tech setting. Trauma surgeons are saving lives but are also attending to weakness, neediness, suffering, and sadness. The empathetic surgeons are also seeing to the invisible wounds that patients carry. Advanced medical care remains a human service provided by humans.

This physical trauma study is in keeping with older studies of persons with mental health problems, where the variability in patient depression outcomes—whether the treatment is pharmacology or psychotherapy—depended on the psychiatrist. The authors proposed that "poor rapport" (another way of saying unkindness) led to ineffective care. Or, to put it another way, there is an implication that the clinician is not only a provider of treatment but also a means of treatment.

A third kind of study again demonstrates that the relational aspects of care are key levers in improving clinical outcomes. This work focuses not on a patient behavior like ED recidivism, or on the long-term consequences after life-saving surgery, but on a simpler medical occasion: an acute illness. Persons coming to a medical office for a common cold were seen by a provider they'd never met before (six doctors were included). Immediately after the visit, the patient answered ten questions that assessed the aspects of the encounter related to what the researchers termed "empathy." Did the doctor make you feel at ease? Allow you to "tell your story"? Take an interest in you as a whole person? Fully understand your concerns? Show care and compassion? For the next fourteen days, patients recorded whether they still believed they had cold symptoms.

Patients who gave their doctor a perfect empathy score had shorter cold durations—nearly a full day—than persons who rated their doctors as less than perfect. Each of the six clinicians in the study saw a comparable proportion of patients reporting perfect empathy scores, precluding the possibility that these results were driven by one clinician being naturally more empathetic than all the others. However, among the two-thirds of patients who gave their clinicians less-than-perfect scores, a higher score—but still one less than perfect—did not predict quicker cold improvement.

So why was the effect seen only among patients who gave their clinicians *perfect* scores? Why was there no relationship of empathy to recovery across the full range of scores—the higher the empathy, the shorter the cold—as one might have predicted? Perhaps this lack of a response to "moderate" levels of empathy tells us something about how patients make judgments during doctor visits. It suggests that the perception of empathy is an on/off phenomenon, such that a patient either feels completely connected to her doctor (a "perfect score") or she doesn't. Wasn't this Veri's lesson? Wasn't this kind of assessment at play when I chose a neurosurgeon?

What is the biological mechanism for perfect empathy shortening cold symptoms? Does empathy inspire optimism or positivity in the patient? Does having someone on your side serve as an antidepressant, and does defusing anxiety simmer down the sympathetic nervous system and lower cortisol? Is trust an immune activator?

The same unsentimental skeptic might accept that kindness can improve how a patient *feels*—after trauma surgery or a cold—but does kindness have an effect on a real, objectively measured medical outcome such as blood pressure?

A final study suggests that kindness might do just this. Two hundred sixty-seven doctors and nurses completed surveys about their empathetic orientation and their sense of burnout. Blood pressure data was obtained from the medical records of the more than 300,000 patients under these providers' care. The researchers made a distinction between adequate and inadequate blood pressure control in accordance with standard guidelines. Here's what they found: patients under the care of physicians with lower self-rated burnout and higher empathy had better blood pressure control overall.

What is the mechanism for this effect, which is seen across a large population of patients, not the few hundred seen in the studies I offered earlier? Hypertension is a condition where both pharmacological (taking one's medications) and nonpharmacological (following medical recommendations about using less salt, or losing weight, or exercising) treatments are important. One could speculate that clinicians who are more empathetic and less burnt out have better verbal and nonverbal communication with patients and spend more time with them, increasing patient satisfaction with care, which in turn leads to better adherence to recommended treatment, which leads to better outcomes. This flow of causation is hypothetical, and of course kindness is not offered to or experienced by each one of these hundreds of thousands of patients. I'm suggesting instead that kindness is felt widely, diffusely, and an effect *on average* is therefore evident, a blood pressure effect that could prevent strokes or heart attacks over the long run.

Across all of these studies, a uniting mechanism might be that under the care of kind doctors, patients have higher expectations of themselves in terms of self-care because they feel heard and valued. Trust in a provider reduces distress so that patients can concentrate, listen more carefully to instructions, and think about themselves more clearly and care-fully when they get home. And at a medical visit, they can talk more about their symptoms and concerns without fear of judgment, allowing the doctor to collect more detailed medical and psychological information to inform better diagnostic and treatment plans.

Kindness matters. But each of these studies has its limitations, as all medical research does. The naysayer can still interject that it would be best to do a randomized trial, our gold standard for scientific proof, to demonstrate that the kinder the doctor, the more successful the patient. But what patient would agree to participate in a study where she might be assigned to an unkind doctor? A slightly less ethically fraught study might select a group of doctors, measure the outcomes of some of their patients (researchers could choose a relatively homogeneous group, perhaps those with medication-treated diabetes) over a period of time, then train the doctors to be more empathetic and measure the outcomes of a second cohort of their diabetic (or hypertensive or asthma) patients going forward (while also measuring the maintenance of the doctors' empathy training effect) to see if these patients do better than the group from before the training. We would predict that those doctors who raised and maintained their empathetic behavior "scores" would have better results than doctors who never improved or let their empathy skills lag. This is a tough, long, and expensive study to perform, requiring a group of doctors willing to participate, an empathy intervention that can truly change doctors' attitudes and abilities, and longitudinal measures of their patients. It's never been done. It also requires a belief that kindness measurably matters.

No one knows if kindness can lower the risk of death or save lives. But it's clear that kindness improves health across a variety of conditions and illnesses.

Kindness is an attitude and a behavior. Attitude is based on moral standards in the mind of the physician that include respect for the patient, interest in him or her, impartiality, receptivity. These standards are formed by a physician's youth and socialization, psychological development, medical training, the contour of a career, personal experience with patients, readings, and peers. Every doctor has a basic willingness to help, but not every one has a genuine interest in and an emphasis on their patient's feelings. Kindness carries with it a commitment to a certain way of thinking and being rather than to a particular predefined endpoint. The best doctors don't even know they're doing it—the benefits of time and talk are unconscious, part of usual care. By showing that they are open to patients' experiences, doctors are helping patients feel better, or at least feel at ease during office visits. We now know they produce better outcomes for chronic conditions, which means they affect the lives of patients outside the office.

There are times when our doctors may be less kind but it matters less to us—when the visit is urgent, when we are in terrible pain and so focused on our bodies we are barely listening as we wait for relief, when we need immediate surgery, when the problem is diagnosed and fixed quickly. A patient's sense of the importance of kindness is always built atop her assumption of her doctor's skill and knowledge. Competence is the sine qua non. Unkindness is never acceptable, but kindness is always what we hope for when we are unwell.

I like to think of kindness as the most natural, easy, obvious, and unremarkable activity in the world. There should be no need for instruction or complaint. It shouldn't need to be outsourced to student volunteers. It's completely reasonable to expect a doctor to be kind at every visit. Yet as a doctor, the idea of a "perfect score" for empathy is terrifying; one wrong move—a gesture, an expression, a few words I might not even know were off-putting—could taint an entire visit.

Perhaps this fear of yet another misstep is why I took time away from work after Beatriz and the two smaller errors that sealed a month of self-critical evaluation. Time off was punishment. I was depriving myself of my great joy, for in my office I am most enmeshed in the lives of others, and where I feel committed and able to express my most generous side. I was saved by meeting two strangers—a doctor and the patient he'd injured. After my visits with them, I began to write this book, which is really the story of my career that followed the loss of my father, my experiences over decades of what I've now come to understand as kindness and unkindness.

The essential experience of illness is loneliness. Feeling alone is the paradoxical essence of our shared humanity. We live in a bubble of one. Each of us feels solitary, and this is made clearest by illness, when we are trapped in a body that betrays us. We are all lonely patients. Kindness is an answer to loneliness, a piercing of loneliness. The affective part of a doctor's work includes recognition of the emotional state and situation of the lonely patient, and being moved by it, recognizing a feeling of identification, even for a moment, with someone who suffers with anger, grief, pain, and disappointment. As my friend Tracy said, "Kindness is letting a patient know that a sad thing has happened."

Kindness, despite the obstacles that may prevent it—the computers that doctors bring into examining rooms to complete the electronic health record, the corporate imposition of fifteen-minute visits, the endless requirement for documentation—is the only way that the medical profession will save itself. Or so I've surmised from my own experiences. My first day of medical school I began my training in unkindness. Nearly forty years after graduation, I heard a story of kindness and forgiveness in a small town near my own that I will never forget. I've reconsidered that old medical school survey question "Would you rather be intelligent or kind?" Kindness is a form of intelligence.

For doctors to do better, the first step is understanding the sources of their unkindness, from their first training as students to the last patient who ignored their advice, to the guilt over the mistakes they make. Kindness is related to tolerance: allowing, indulging, and enduring what a patient brings forth. It is not a solution to a specific problem, but a signal of curiosity about a patient's suffering. Kindness must be active, and it describes not the relationship between healer and healed but a covenant between equals, one of whom needs helps in the moment. Kindness is part of the contract every doctor signs when she agrees to meet with a patient, and she must hold herself to it.

But we often forget that doctors, too, are often in need of forgiveness—from their patients and from themselves. No doctor enters the medical profession expecting to be unkind or make mistakes, yet because of the complexity of our current medical system, and because doctors are as fallible as other humans, we often find ourselves acting much less kindly than we would like to. Patients want relief from self-blame; doctors do too. We are all looking for ways to forgive ourselves.

Medicine has until recently remained one of the constant bastions of kindness, and the doctor a figure of benign authority, an inspiration, the embodiment of kindness. I want to revive the model of the doctor as the instantiation of kindness. I want a romantic rebirth in my profession. Kindness in the office, the clinic, the emergency room, the hospital, the medical world, must serve as an exemplar for kindness in the wider world.

ACKNOWLEDGMENTS

These essays were written over many years and helped along by the kindnesses of extraordinary people. My dear friend Michael Lowenthal, the clearest thinker and sharpest editor, reshaped each one of these pieces, and let me keep asking questions until the final word was settled. His time and mind were great gifts. The editors of the magazines that published pieces collected here—William Pierce and Sven Birkerts at *Agni*, Willard Spiegelman when he was at *Southwest Review*, Christina Thompson at *Harvard Review*, and staff at the *Washington Post*—offered great first homes for this writing. I'm grateful to the editors of the Best American Essays Series who selected some of these chapters as notables.

Doctor friends Michele Cyr, Bill Tsiaris, and Trish Cioe told me stories from their own daily rounds with humor and modesty. Carol Landau thought this book's topic was worth pursuing, gave me confidence to pursue it, and never giggled when I ordered hot chocolate after she ordered coffee during our morning discussions. Jeffrey Samet and Marc Gourevich remain the steadiest and most supportive voices in my medical ear, their own work an inspiration. My walking and talking partner for decades, Peter Kramer, heard me jabber on and second-guess far too much, and then gave me books to read to simmer me down before our next stroll.

Huge thanks to the team at University of North Carolina Press for their joyous care: Dino Battista, Liz Orange, Sonya Bonczek, Mary Caviness; they are all a pleasure to work with. Most of all I'm grateful to my editor and shepherd Lucas Church, who welcomed me aboard and kept me on track.

I've seen thousands of patients over the years, and thought about them thousands of nights. Many I've gotten to know well and cared for over decades—long enough that one of my favorites recently said, "When I met you, I was dying, and you had hair. Now you're bald and I'm doing just fine." I owe special thanks to the real Ms. P and Dr. S, both wounded, whom I met by chance and who let me into their lives, generously spoke with me for hours about their pasts and feelings about how care goes wrong and then right, and provided me with the lessons of forgiveness.

To my first and closest reader, Hester, who has forgiven.

REFERENCES

Chapter 1

Dinsmore, Charles E., Steven Daugherty, and Howard J. Zeitz. "Student Responses to the Gross Anatomy Laboratory in a Medical Curriculum." *Clinical Anatomy* 14, no. 3 (2001): 231–36. https://doi .org/10.1002/ca.1038.

Finkelstein, Peter, and Lawrence H. Mathers. "Post-traumatic Stress among Medical Students in the Anatomy Dissection Laboratory." *Clinical Anatomy* 3 (1990): 219–26. https://doi.org/10.1002 /ca.980030308.

Goebert, Deborah, Diane Thompson, Junji Takeshita, Cheryl Beach, Philip Bryson, Kimberly Ephgrave, Alan Kent, Monique Kunkel, Joel Schechter, and Jodi Tate. "Depressive Symptoms in Medical Students and Residents: A Multischool Study." *Academic Medicine* 84, no. 2 (2009): 236–41. https://doi.org/10.1097 /ACM.0b013e31819391bb.

Hafferty, Frederic W. *Into the Valley: Death and the Socialization of Medical Students*. New Haven, Conn.: Yale University Press, 1991.

Hojat, Mohammadreza, Michael J. Vergare, Kaye Maxwell, George C. Brainard, Steven K. Herrine, Gerald A. Isenberg, John Veloski, and Joseph S. Gonnella. "The Devil Is in the Third Year: A Longitudinal Study of Erosion of Empathy in Medical School." *Academic Medicine* 84, no. 9 (2009): 1182–91. https://doi.org/10.1097/ACM.0b013e3181b17e55.

Marks, Sandy C., Jr., Sandra L. Bertman, and June C. Penney. "Human Anatomy: A Foundation for Education about Death and Dying in Medicine." *Clinical Anatomy* 10, no. 2 (1997): 118–22. https://doi .org/10.1002/(SICI)1098-2353(1997)10:2<118::AID-CA8>3.0 .CO;2-R.

McGarvey, Alice, T. Farrell, Ronán Michael Conroy, and S. Kandiah. "Dissection: A Positive Experience." *Clinical Anatomy* 14 (2001): 227–30. https://doi.org/10.1002/ca.1037.

Peterson, Cora, Aaron Sussell, Jia Li, Pamelia K. Schumacher, Kristin Yeoman, and Deborah M. Stone. "Suicide Rates by Industry and Occupation—National Violent Death Reporting System, 32 States, 2016." *MMWR—Morbidity and Mortality Weekly Report* 69, no. 3 (2020): 57–62. https://doi.org/10.15585/mmwr .mm6903a1.

Wegner, Daniel M., David J. Schneider, Samuel R. Carter, and Teri L. White. "Paradoxical Effects of Thought Suppression." *Journal of Personality and Social Psychology* 53, no. 1 (1987): 5–13. https://doi .org/10.1037//0022-3514.53.1.5.

Chapter 2

Baumeister, Roy F., Ellen Bratslavsky, Mark Muraven, and Dianne M. Tice. "Ego Depletion: Is the Active Self a Limited Resource?" *Journal of Personality and Social Psychology* 74, no. 5 (1998): 1252–65. https://doi.org/10.1037//0022-3514.74.5.1252.

Baumeister, Roy F., Kathleen D. Vohs, and Dianne M. Tice. "The Strength Model of Self-Control." *Current Directions in Psychological Science* 16, no. 6 (2007): 351–55. https://doi .org/10.1111/j.1467-8721.2007.00534.x.

Inzlicht, Michael, Brandon J. Schmeichel, and C. Neil Macrae. "Why Self-Control Seems (but May Not Be) Limited." *Trends Cognitive Sciences* 18, no. 3 (2014): 127–33. https://doi.org/10.1016/j .tics.2013.12.009.

Chapter 3

Fogarty, Linda A., Barbara A. Curbow, John R. Wingard, Karen McDonnell, and Mark R. Somerfield. "Can 40 Seconds of Compassion Reduce Patient Anxiety?" *Journal of Clinical Oncology* 17, no. 1 (1999): 371–79. https://doi.org/10.1200/JCO.1999.17.1.371.

Parsons, Talcott. *The Social System.* Glencoe, Ill.: Free Press, 1964.

Chapter 4

Cheng, Yawei, Ching-Po Lin, Ho-Ling Liu, Yuan-Yu Hsu, Kun-Eng Lim, Daisy Hung, and Jean Decety. "Expertise Modulates the Perception of Pain in Others." *Current Biology* 17, no. 19 (2007): 1708–13. https://doi.org/10.1016/j.cub.2007.09.020.

Danziger, Nicolas, Kenneth M. Prkachin, and Jean-Claude Willer. "Is Pain the Price of Empathy? The Perception of Others' Pain in Patients with Congenital Insensitivity to Pain." *Brain* 129, part 9 (2006): 2494–2507. https://doi.org/10.1093/brain/awl155.

Decety, Jean, and Yoshiya Moriguchi. "The Empathic Brain and Its Dysfunction in Psychiatric Populations: Implications for Intervention across Different Clinical Conditions." *Biopsychosocial Medicine* 1 (2007): 22. https://doi.org/10.1186/1751-0759-1-22.

Figley, Charles R. "Compassion Fatigue: Psychotherapists' Chronic Lack of Self Care." *Journal of Clinical Psychology* 58, no. 11 (2002): 1433–41. https://doi.org/10.1002/jclp.10090.

Joinson, Carla. "Coping with Compassion Fatigue." *Nursing* 22, no. 4 (1992): 118–19. PMID: 1570090.

Lamm, Claus, C. Daniel Batson, and Jean Decety. "The Neural Substrate of Human Empathy: Effects of Perspective-Taking and Cognitive Appraisal." *Journal of Cognitive Neuroscience* 19, no. 1 (2007): 42–58. https://doi.org/10.1162/jocn.2007.19.1.42.

Maslach, Christina, and Susan E. Jackson. "The Measurement of Experienced Burnout." *Journal of Occupational Behaviour* 2 (1981): 99–113. https://doi.org/10.1002/JOB.4030020205.

Schulz, Richard, Randy S. Hebert, Mary Amanda Dew, Stephanie L. Brown, Michael F. Scheier, Scott R. Beach, Sara J. Czaja, Lynn M. Martire, David Coon, Kenneth M. Langa, Laura N. Gitlin, Alan B. Stevens, and Linda Nichols. "Patient Suffering and Caregiver Compassion: New Opportunities for Research, Practice, and Policy." *Gerontologist* 47, no. 1 (2007): 4–13. https://doi.org/10.1093/geront/47.1.4.

Chapter 5

Ambady, Nalini. "The Perils of Pondering: Intuition and Thin Slice Judgments." *Psychological Inquiry* 21, no. 4 (2010): 271–78. https://doi.org/10.1080/1047840X.2010.524882.

Ambady, Nalini, and Heather M. Gray. "On Being Sad and Mistaken: Mood Effects on the Accuracy of Thin-Slice Judgments." *Journal of Personality and Social Psychology* 83, no. 4 (2002): 947–61. PMID: 12374446.

Ambady, Nalini, Debi LaPlante, Thai Nguyen, Robert Rosenthal, Nigel Chaumeton, and Wendy Levinson. "Surgeons' Tone of Voice: A Clue to Malpractice History." *Surgery* 132, no. 1 (2002): 5–9. https://doi.org/10.1067/msy.2002.124733.

Chapter 9

Blendon, Robert J., Catherine M. DesRoches, Mollyann Brodie, John M. Benson, Allison B. Rosen, Eric Schneider, Drew E. Altman, Kinga Zapert, Melissa J. Herrmann, and Annie E. Steffenson. "Views of Practicing Physicians and the Public on Medical Errors." *New England Journal of Medicine* 347, no. 24 (2002): 1933–40. https://doi.org/10.1056/NEJMsa022151.

Griswold, Charles. *Forgiveness: A Philosophical Exploration*. Cambridge: Cambridge University Press, 2007.

Levinson, Wendy, and Nigel Chaumeton. "Communication between Surgeons and Patients in Routine Office Visits." *Surgery* 125, no. 2 (1999): 127–34. PMID: 10026744.

Levinson, Wendy, Debra L. Roter, John P. Mullooly, Valerie T. Dull, and Richard M. Frankel. "Physician-Patient Communication: The Relationship with Malpractice Claims among Primary Care Physicians and Surgeons." *JAMA—Journal of the American Medical Association* 277, no. 7 (1997): 553–59. https://doi.org/10.1001/jama.277.7.553p.

Studdert, David M., Eric J. Thomas, Helen R. Burstin, Brett I. W. Zbar, E. John Orav, and Troyen A. Brennan. "Negligent Care and Malpractice Claiming Behavior in Utah and Colorado." *Medical Care* 38, no. 3 (2000): 250–60. https://doi.org/10.1097/00005650-200003000 -00002.

Tai-Seale, Ming, Thomas G. McGuire, and Weimin Zhang. "Time Allocation in Primary Care Office Visits." *Health Services Research* 42, no. 5 (2007): 1871–94. https://doi.org/10.1111/j.1475-6773.2006.00689.x.

Wu, Albert W., I.-Chan Huang, Samantha Stokes, and Peter J. Provonost. "Disclosing Medical Errors to Patients: It's Not What You Say, It's What They Hear." *Journal of General Internal Medicine* 24, no. 9 (2009): 1012–17. https://doi.org/10.1007/s11606-009-1044-3.

Chapter 10

Chaitoff, Alexander, Michael B. Rothberg, Amy K. Windover, Leonard Calabrese, Amita D. Misra-Hebert, and Kathryn A. Martinez. "Physician Empathy Is Not Associated with Laboratory Outcomes in Diabetes: A Cross-Sectional Study." *Journal of General Internal Medicine* 34, no. 1 (2019): 75–81. https://doi.org/10.1007 /s11606018-4731-0.

Del Canale, Stefano, Daniel Z. Louis, Vittorio Maio, Xiaohong Wang, Giuseppina Rossi, Mohammedreza Hojat, and Joseph S. Gonella. "The Relationship between Physician Empathy and Disease Complications: An Empirical Study of Primary Care Physicians and

Their Diabetic Patients in Parma, Italy." *Academic Medicine* 87, no. 9 (2012): 1243–49. https://doi.org/10.1097/ACM.0b013e3182628fbf.

Kelley, John M., Gordon Kraft-Todd, Lidia Schapira, Joe Kossowsky, and Helen Riess. "The Influence of the Patient-Clinician Relationship on Healthcare Outcomes: A Systematic Review and Meta-Analysis of Randomized Controlled Trials." *PLoS One* 9, no. 4 (2014): e94207. https://doi.org/10.1371/journal.pone.0094207.

Rakel, David, Bruce Barrett, Zhengjun Zhang, Theresa Hoeft, Betty Chewning, Lucille Marchand, and Jo Scheder. "Perception of Empathy in the Therapeutic Encounter: Effects on the Common Cold." *Patient Education and Counseling* 85, no. 3 (2011): 390–97. https://doi.org/10.1016/j.pec.2011.01.009.

Stein, Michael. *The Lonely Patient: How We Experience Illness.* New York: William Morrow, 2007.

Steinhausen, Simone, Oliver Ommen, Sonja Thüm, Rolf Lefering, Thorsten Koehler, Edmund Neugebauer, and Holger Pfaff. "Physician Empathy and Subjective Evaluation of Medical Treatment Outcome in Trauma Surgery Patients." *Patient Education and Counseling* 95, no. 1 (2014): 53–60. https://doi.org/10.1016/j.pec.2013.12.007.

Yuguero, Oriol, Josep Ramon Marsal, Montserrat Esquerda, and Jorge Soler-González. "Occupational Burnout and Empathy Influence Blood Pressure Control in Primary Care Physicians." *BMC Family Practice* 18, no. 1 (2017): 63. https://doi.org/10.1186/s12875-017-0634-0.